Renal Wellness Kitchen

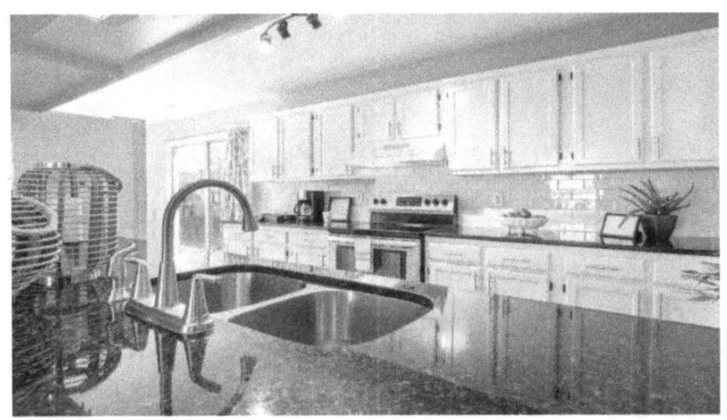

A Comprehensive Guide to Kidney-Boosting Recipes for Optimal Health

JANICE M. REESE

TABLE OF CONTENT

INTRODUCTION

Sarah, a lively neighbor in her early forties, lived next door to me. Her garden was the talk of the neighborhood, and her laughter used to fill it. However, when she received the renal illness diagnosis, her life unexpectedly changed.

Sarah's previously hectic life started to take a toll due to her health issues. Her laughing got muted and the beautiful garden she lovingly cared began to wither. The regimented renal diet, with its strange limitations, towered over her.

However, Sarah was never one to back down from a fight. She set out on her quest for improved health with unyielding resolve. She adopted the renal diet with her family's help and her renewed determination.

The shift started to become apparent gradually. Sarah discovered how to appreciate the inherent tastes of in-season, low-potassium fruits and vegetables. She found that flavorings such as parsley, basil, and oregano may add depth to her food without adding too much salt. Her family came to cook with her, trying out new recipes and coming up with kidney-friendly meals that were as tasty as they were healthful.

Months passed, and Sarah's perseverance paid off. Her vitality restored, her renal function normalized, and her health started to recover. She spent time outside caring to her cherished plants, and her garden - which had been neglected - began to bloom once more.

Sarah started getting back in touch with her hobbies with her renewed energy. She brought friends around for boisterous get-togethers, offering delectable kidney-friendly foods that left everyone amazed. Once again, the community was united and joyful by Sarah's laughing.

Her journey from a state of uncertainty to one of restored health and happiness served as a testimonial to the transformational potential of the renal diet. Sarah's life, which had previously been shadowed by her health issues, now shone with the warmth of her laughter and the vivid colors of her garden, showing us all that one can rediscover life's joys even in the midst of hardship if they have perseverance and support.

CHAPTER ONE

Your Kitchen, Your Haven

- Putting Kidney-Friendly Magic on the Shelves

One of the most important parts of eating a renal diet to support kidney health is stocking the shelves with Kidney-Friendly Magic. By taking this step, you can make sure that you always have the correct components on hand to make satisfying meals that follow your dietary requirements.

1. *Fresh Produce:* Stock your refrigerator and pantry with an assortment of fresh, low-potassium fruits and vegetables to start. Select produce such as green beans, cabbage, cauliflower, apples, berries, and grapes. These choices supply vital nutrients without unduly taxing the kidneys.

2. *Lean Proteins:* Provide space for protein sources that are good for your kidneys. Egg whites, salmon, and skinless chicken are good sources of lean meat. Legumes like lentils and chickpeas, as well as plant-based proteins like tofu, are other options.

3. *Whole Grains:* Make sure you consume enough of whole grains, such as whole wheat pasta, quinoa, and brown rice.

When compared to their refined equivalents, these grains have less phosphorus.

4. ***Dairy Substitutes:*** Keep calcium-fortified non-dairy milk substitutes like almond, rice, or oat milk on hand if you're on a renal diet that excludes dairy products.

5. ***Low-Sodium Broths:*** Choose homemade broths that are created with fresh ingredients or low-sodium broths. These can serve as the foundation for many cuisines, such as stews and soups.

6. ***Veggies, both canned and frozen:*** Stock your cupboard with a variety of low-sodium or no-salt-added canned and frozen veggies. These are easy to prepare and suitable for kidneys.

7. ***Herbs & Spices:*** These are your go-to tools for flavor addition when you don't want to use too much salt. Add a range of seasonings that are healthy for kidneys, such as garlic powder, thyme, basil, and oregano.

8. ***Low-Phosphorus Foods:*** Be mindful of the amount of phosphorus in the products in your cupboard. Seek for low-phosphorus substitutes, such as low-phosphorus baking flour and cereals made with rice.

9. ***Heart-healthy Oils:*** For cooking and salad dressings, use heart-healthy oils like olive oil. These oils are healthier for kidney health since they contain less saturated fat.

10. ***Limit High-Potassium Ingredients:*** Take care to avoid high-potassium foods like potatoes, tomatoes, and bananas when restocking your shelves. If your diet permits, keep them as a treat or in moderation.

11. ***Read Labels:*** Make sure you always read nutrition labels to find out how much phosphorus, potassium, and sodium are in packaged goods. Choose products that have fewer of these minerals in them.

12. ***Plan and Organize:*** Lastly, make sure you have all the kidney-friendly items you need for your weekly meals by planning your meals and creating shopping lists ahead of time.

- Prepare Yourself for Success in the Kitchen

Welcome to the realm of renal nutrition, where you may enjoy the delicious and fulfilling benefits of maintaining the health of your kidneys. A good chef has to have the correct kitchenware, just as an accomplished painter has the best brushes and paints. We'll walk you through stocking your kitchen with the necessities for your renal diet journey in this section.

- Essentials of Cooking: Your Kitchen Must-Haves

Make a special section in your cookbook with a list and explanation of all the ingredients needed in cooking.

- Invest in high-quality cookware, such as oven-safe bakeware, stainless steel pots, and non-stick pans. These can help you achieve your nutritional objectives by reducing the amount of fat and oil you use in your cooking while also increasing cooking efficiency.

- *Sharp Knives:* Your reliable kitchen partner is a pair of well-made, razor-sharpened knives. They make sure your kidney-friendly items are chopped, sliced, and chopped safely and precisely.

- *Cutting boards:* Choose easy-to-clean materials like plastic or bamboo to reduce the possibility of cross-contamination. When incorporating different components into a renal diet, this is essential.

- *Measuring Cups and Spoons:* The key to a successful renal diet is precise measuring. To measure ingredients precisely and monitor your nutrient intake, use a sturdy set of measuring cups and spoons.

- Food processors and blenders are multipurpose kitchen tools that let you make sauces, purees, and smoothies from scratch and cut down on packaged foods high in salt.

- *Digital Kitchen Scale:* For accurate weight measurements, a kitchen scale is your hidden weapon. This is especially helpful if you have strict dietary restrictions.

- *Vegetable Peeler and Grater:* Use these tools to make preparing fruits and vegetables easier and to improve the taste and texture of your food.

- Vegetables retain their original tastes and nutrients when steamed rather than cooked, thus a steamer is a vital kitchen appliance for kidney-friendly cooking.

- *Slow Cooker:* With little effort, a slow cooker makes it easier to prepare foods that need for lengthy, slow cooking times. Ideal for days when you're busy on your renal diet journey.

- ***Instant-Read Thermometer:*** Use an instant-read thermometer to monitor the temperature of meats and poultry to ensure the safety and quality of your dishes.

- ***Citrus Juicer:*** Savor the flavor of fresh citrus fruits as a tasty, low-sodium way to add flair to your meals.

- ***Salad Spinner:*** Rinse and dry leafy greens and herbs with a salad spinner to keep your salads crisp and fresh.

- ***Sieve or strainer:*** To lower the salt level of canned vegetables and beans, drain and rinse them well.

- ***Cooking Utensils:*** Choose silicone or wooden utensils that won't damage non-stick surfaces or be rough on your cookware.

- ***Storage Containers:*** To maintain freshness and avoid cross-contamination of flavors, use a range of airtight containers to store preparing components and leftovers.

Your kitchen is your sanctuary and these necessities are your allies as you go on a gastronomic adventure through the realm of renal diet. With the correct resources and information at your disposal, you may take proactive measures to maintain the health of your kidneys in addition to cooking delicious meals. So stock your kitchen, take charge of your life, and let's go on this tasty and fulfilling renal diet journey together.

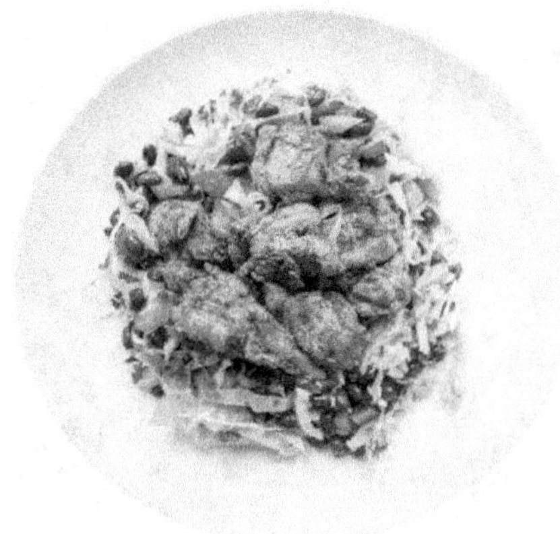

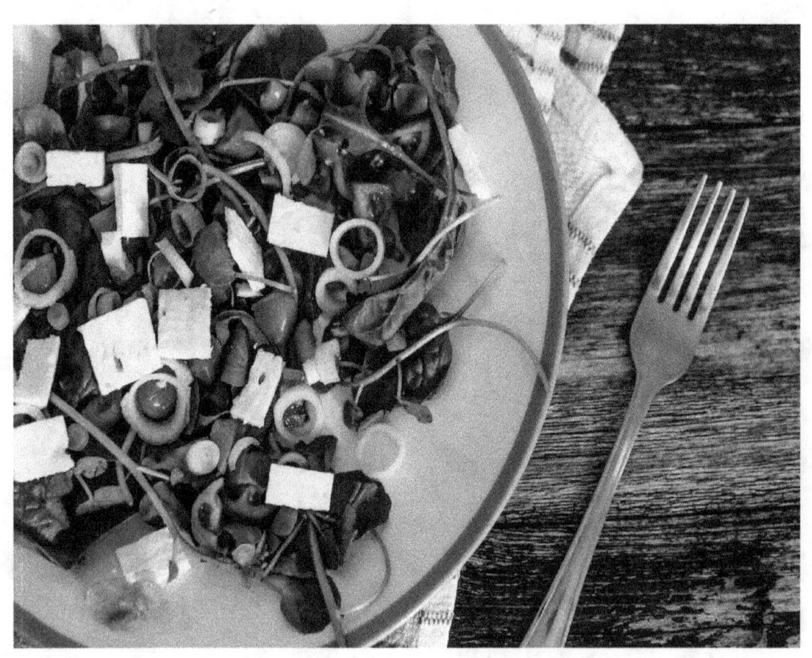

CHAPTER TWO

Learning the Fundamentals of the Renal Diet

- Macronutrients and Micronutrients: The Symphony of Nutrients

Knowing how to balance macro and micronutrients in a renal diet is like playing a beautiful symphony. The same way that a trained conductor arranges different instruments to produce beautiful music, we too need to arrange the correct nutrients to maintain kidney function and general wellbeing.

Macronutrients: The Building Blocks of Your Harmony

1. *Protein:* Consider protein to be the foundation of your nutritional composition. Protein is necessary for development, repair, and general health, but those with renal problems need to watch how much they eat. The melody is provided without taxing your kidneys by high-quality, low-phosphorus foods such lean meats, poultry, fish, and plant-based alternatives like tofu and lentils.

2. *Carbohydrates:* Your nutritional symphony has rhythm and energy thanks to carbohydrates. Choose complex carbs, such as those found in whole grains, fruits, and vegetables, since they provide a continuous energy source and important fiber without causing blood sugar levels to rise.

3. *Fats:* The richness and depth of your diet are enhanced by fats. The velvety undertones that give your meals a heart-healthy, gratifying flavor are provided by heart-healthy fats like those in almonds, avocados, and olive oil.

Micronutrients: Your Symphony's Finer Notes

1. *Sodium:* Providing structure and balance, sodium is comparable to the percussion section. Limiting salt consumption is essential on a renal diet to preserve blood pressure and appropriate fluid balance. To control sodium, season your food with herbs, spices, and low-sodium substitutes.

2. *Potassium:* Like the string section, potassium is delicately involved in the function of muscles and nerves. However, too much potassium can be dangerous for those who have renal problems. By selecting fruits and vegetables low in

potassium and according to your healthcare provider's advice, you may keep the proper balance.

3. ***Phosphorus:*** The brass part, phosphorus is necessary for the health of bones and the synthesis of energy. Because the kidneys have trouble regulating phosphorus, avoid high-phosphorus foods such as dairy, processed meats, and sodas. Accept low-phosphorus foods for a balanced diet.

4. ***Calcium:*** The woodwind part, calcium is necessary for heart and bone health. Calcium supplements are a common part of a renal diet, which helps you achieve your needs while controlling your phosphorus levels.

5. ***Vitamins and Minerals:*** Vitamins and minerals are the soloists, each with a distinct role, much like the many instruments in a symphony. Iron, vitamin C, and B vitamins are all important nutrients to have in your diet. Make sure you obtain these nutrients via kidney-friendly foods, supplements, or prescription drugs.

- Symphony Balancing: Your Dietary Conductor

You are the conductor of your own nutritional symphony when it comes to renal nutrition. To make sure your diet is tailored to your unique needs, it's critical to collaborate closely with your healthcare practitioner or dietitian. Your tools for creating a balanced and kidney-friendly diet include blood tests, regular check-ups, and dietary changes.

Therefore, when you begin your renal diet journey, see your meals as musical compositions and keep in mind that a dietary symphony that is both beautiful and health-promoting may be created with the correct ratio of macronutrients to micronutrients.

- Controlling the Trio: Phosphorus, Sodium, and Potassium

- Sodium: The Harmony of Equilibrium

- Consider salt to be the orchestra's rhythm section in your diet. It's essential for preserving fluid equilibrium as well as healthy neuron and muscle function. However, if consumed in excess, it can cause fluid retention and high blood pressure, both of which can put strain on your kidneys. Controlling sodium entails:

- Examining food labels to find substances in packaged foods that are high in salt.

- Making meals from scratch to reduce the amount of salt.

- Seasoning your food with herbs, spices, and low-sodium substitutes.

- Potassium: The Controlling Melody

Potassium has a critical role in the function of muscles and nerves. But too much potassium can upset this balance and perhaps cause damage to your heart and muscles. Controlling potassium:

- Select fruits and vegetables that are low in potassium, such as green beans, apples, and berries.

- Recognize and limit your intake of foods high in potassium, such as tomatoes and bananas.

- Track your potassium levels with routine blood testing.

Phosphorus: The Balance of Harmony

- Phosphorus gives your diet the harmonic depth that is necessary for the health of your bones and the synthesis of energy. Your body may find it difficult to control phosphorus levels if you have renal difficulties, which can result in bone disorders and other health concerns. Controlling phosphorus entails:

- Reducing consumption of foods rich in phosphorus, such as dairy, processed meats, and sodas.

- Adopting low-phosphorus substitutes such as cereals made of rice and utilizing phosphorus binders in accordance with physician prescriptions.

- Closely collaborating with your medical team to track your phosphorus levels and modify your diet as necessary.

- Moving Through the Wet Landscape: Managing Fluids

Managing fluid intake in the context of renal nutrition is similar to navigating a muddy terrain. You may learn to direct your fluid intake to promote kidney health and general well-being, just like a good captain does while navigating the waters.

- The Challenge: Balancing Act

Fluids are essential for keeping the kidneys healthy. They support the kidneys in controlling bodily processes and removing waste. It takes a delicate balance, nevertheless, to properly regulate fluids for people with renal problems. While drinking too little might result in dehydration, consuming too much can promote fluid retention and elevated blood pressure.

- ***Know Your Limits:*** Determine your daily fluid limit in close consultation with your physician or nutritionist. It's imperative that you adhere to this restriction strictly because it's tailored to your unique situation.

- ***Monitor Your Thirst:*** Take note of your body's cues and sip as it becomes necessary. Refrain from overindulging in alcohol owing to habits or meals that cause dehydration.

- ***Regulate Your Fluid Intake:*** Pay attention to the liquids that are concealed in meals like soups, fruits, and vegetables in addition to what you drink. These are deducted from your daily cap.

Fluid Substitutes: Ingenious Remedies

Even if fluid management might be difficult, there are inventive solutions to enhance your experience:

- ***Restrict Rich-Fluid Foods:*** Cucumbers and watermelon are two examples of foods rich in water content. You may better manage your fluid consumption by consuming these meals in moderation.

- ***Chew Gum or Suck on Ice Chips:*** You can treat dry mouth without drinking more water by chewing sugar-free gum or sucking on ice chips.

- ***Remain Cool and Refreshed:*** To remain cool on hot days, use a fan or a spray bottle. By doing this, you can lessen your thirst without consuming additional liquids.

Observing and Modifying: Your Guidance Instruments

Your dietician and healthcare professional are your guides when it comes to fluid management. Regular check-ups and blood tests will be used to track your progress, and they will change your fluid restriction as necessary. You may overcome this hurdle and protect the health of your kidneys by following your prescribed fluid restriction, keeping an eye on your thirst, and making thoughtful decisions.

CHAPTER THREE

Dawn Delights: Kidney-Friendly Breakfasts

- Magic Mornings with Low-Potassium Choices

- Spiced oatmeal topped with quickly stewed apples

Ingredients:

For Spiced Porridge:

- Half a cup of steel-cut oats

- Half a cup of water

- Half a cup of low-potassium milk, like rice or almond milk

- Half a teaspoon of cinnamon, ground

- 1/4 teaspoon of nutmeg, ground

- To taste, 1 tablespoon honey or sugar substitute

- An optional pinch of salt

For Quick-Stewed Apples:

- One apple (choose a Granny Smith or other low-potassium kind).

- 1/4 teaspoon of cinnamon powder

- Half a spoonful of honey or an alternative sugar

Instructions:

1. **Prepare the Quick-Stewed Apples:**

- Clean the apple and peel it. Slice the core into thin, tiny pieces after removing it.

- Place the apple slices and a tiny amount of water in a small pot.

- Sprinkle the apples with ground cinnamon and sweeten with honey or a sugar alternative (adjust sweetness to your desire).

- Simmer the apples for 5 to 7 minutes, stirring now and again, over low heat, or until they are soft and beginning to caramelize. Take off the heat and place aside.

2. **Get the Porridge Spiced Ready:**

- Boil one and a half cups of water in a different pan.

- Turn down the heat and stir in the steel-cut oats. Cook, stirring periodically, until the oats are creamy and cooked to your preferred consistency, 20 to 25 minutes.

- Stir in the low-potassium milk, ground nutmeg, cinnamon, and honey (or sugar substitute), and season with salt to taste. Simmer for a further two to three minutes to let the flavors combine and the porridge thicken.

3. **Serve:**

- Transfer the spiced oatmeal to a bowl using a spoon.

- Place the quickly stewed apples on top of the oatmeal.

Estimated Preparation Time:

The preparation of this Spiced Porridge with Quick-Stewed Apples takes around thirty minutes.

Nutritional Value (approximately, for one serving):

- 250-300 calories

- 4–6 grams of protein

- 6 to 8 grams of fiber

- Potassium: 100–200 mg (may differ depending on apple variety and kind of low-potassium milk used).

- 100–150 mg of phosphorus

- Sodium: Changes according to salt addition

- Sugar: 10–15 grams (may differ according on kind and quantity of sweetener added)

- Toast with creamy garlic beans

Ingredients:

- 1 can (15 ounces) of washed and drained low-sodium white beans (cannellini or navy beans).

- Two minced garlic cloves

- 1/4 cup veggie broth with reduced sodium

- Two tablespoons of low-potassium milk (rice or almond milk, for example).

- 1/2 teaspoon of dried thyme (or sprigs of fresh thyme)

- To taste, add salt and pepper.

- Two slices of whole-grain bread (choose one with reduced salt content).

- One tablespoon of finely chopped fresh parsley (for garnish)

- One teaspoon olive oil (optional for toasting the bread)

Instructions:

1. Get the creamy garlicky beans ready:

- Heat the minced garlic in a nonstick pan over low heat for one minute, just until fragrant but not browned.

- Stir in the garlic after adding the washed and drained white beans to the skillet.

2. Let the beans cook:

- Add the low-potassium milk and low-sodium vegetable broth.

- Add the salt, pepper, and dried or fresh thyme leaves, according to taste.

- Simmer the beans for five to seven minutes over medium heat, letting the liquid evaporate and the beans get tender and flavorful.

3. Let the bread toast:

- Toast the pieces of whole-grain bread while the beans are cooking. Toasted or pan-toasted till golden brown, you can also toss them with a little coat of olive oil.

4. Serve:

- Transfer the toast to a platter.

- Drizzle the bread with the creamy garlic beans.

- For a pop of freshness, sprinkle freshly chopped parsley on top.

Estimated Preparation Time:

The preparation time for this Creamy Garlic Beans on Toast dish is about 15 to 20 minutes.

Nutritional Value (approximately, for one serving):

- 250 and 300 calories

- 10–12 grams of protein

- 8–10 grams of fiber

- 200–250 milligrams of potassium

- 150–200 mg of phosphorus

- Sodium: varies according on the particular low-sodium components that are utilized.

- **Wholegrain muffins with blueberries**

Ingredients:

– One cup flour, whole wheat

- 1/2 cup of oat flour (create your own by blending rolled oats)

- 1/4 cup erythritol or Stevia, or another sugar alternative

- One and a half tsp baking powder

- One-half tsp baking soda

- 1/4 tsp salt (if using)

- Half a cup of plain applesauce

- 1/4 cup rice or almond milk, or other low-potassium milk

- Two tsp olive oil

- One big egg, or an alternative egg

- One tsp vanilla essence

- One cup low-potassium blueberries, either fresh or frozen

Instructions:

1. Get ready and warm up:

- Set the oven temperature to 175°C, or 350°F.

- To avoid sticking, gently oil the muffin cups or line a muffin tray with paper liners.

2. Blend the Dry Elements:

- Combine the whole wheat flour, oat flour, sugar replacement, baking soda, baking powder, and salt (if using) in a large mixing basin. Make careful to mix them well.

3. Mix Wet Ingredients:

- Combine the unsweetened applesauce, olive oil, low-potassium milk, egg (or egg substitute), and vanilla extract in a another bowl. Blend the ingredients until it's well-blended and smooth.

4. Integrate the Dry and Wet Mixtures:

- Gently incorporate the dry ingredients into the liquid components after pouring them in. Mix just enough to moisten the dry ingredients; take care not to overmix.

5. Add the blueberries

- Fold in the blueberries gently. Don't defrost frozen blueberries before adding them.

6. Stuff muffin liners:

- Evenly distribute the muffin batter among the lined muffin cups, filling each to approximately two-thirds of the way.

7. Bake:

- Bake for 20 to 25 minutes in a preheated oven, or until a toothpick inserted into the middle comes out clean and the muffins are golden brown.

8. Relax and have fun:

- After a few minutes of cooling in the muffin pan, move the muffins to a wire rack to finish cooling.

Estimated Preparation Time:

With baking time, this recipe for Blueberry Wholegrain Muffins takes around 30 to 35 minutes.

Nutritional Value (about, per muffin):

- 100 and 120 calories

- 3–4 grams of protein

- 2–3 grams of fiber

- 50–70 mg of potassium

- 50–70 mg of phosphorus

- Sodium: varies according on the particular low-sodium components that are utilized.

The nutritional contents of any dish for the renal diet may change depending on the brands and products you choose. Tailor this recipe to your own dietary requirements.

- Goat cheese and spring onions atop an omelette

Ingredients:

- Two big eggs

- Two tablespoons of low-potassium milk (rice or almond milk, for example).

- Two spring onions, or green onions, cut finely

- One ounce (28 grams) of crumbled goat cheese

- 1/4 teaspoon of pepper, black

- 1/4 tsp salt (if using)

- One teaspoon of cooking olive oil

Instructions:

1. Get the eggs ready:

- Crack the eggs into a bowl, then whisk in the low-potassium milk. Beat until thoroughly blended. If preferred, add salt and black pepper for seasoning. Put away.

2. Cook the Onions for Spring:

- Heat the olive oil in a nonstick pan over medium-low heat. Add the chopped spring onions and sauté for two to three minutes, or until they start to turn translucent and become soft.

3. Pour the Egg Mixture:

- Cover the skillet's sautéed spring onions with the beaten egg mixture.

4. **Prepare the omelet:** Give the omelette a few minutes to cook without interacting. Using a spatula, carefully raise the edges as they harden to let the raw eggs run below.

5. **Blend in goat cheese:** Evenly scatter the crumbled goat's cheese over half of the omelette when it's almost set but still somewhat runny in the center.

6. Serve:

- Gently fold the remaining omelette in half over the cheese to form a half-moon.

- Simmer for one more minute, or until the cheese starts to melt.

- Transfer the omelette to a platter and, if you wish, top with additional finely chopped spring onions.

Estimated Preparation Time:

The preparation of this dish for Omelet with Spring Onions and Goat's Cheese takes around ten to fifteen minutes.

Nutritional Value (approximately, for one omelette):

- 250 and 300 calories

- 15–17 grams of protein

- 150–200 milligrams of potassium

- 120–150 mg of phosphorus

- Sodium: Changes according to salt addition

- **Cranberries and macadamia nuts with buckwheat granola**

Ingredients:

- One cup uncooked buckwheat groats

- 1/2 cup chopped unsalted macadamia nuts - 1/2 cup dried cranberries (be sure to get ones without extra potassium)

- 1/2 teaspoon ground cinnamon - 1/4 cup unsweetened shredded coconut - 2 tablespoons honey or sugar alternative - 1 tablespoon olive oil

- An optional pinch of salt

Instructions:

1. **Get ready and warm up:**

 - Set the oven's temperature to 325°F (163°C).

- To avoid sticking, line a baking sheet with silicone baking mats or parchment paper.

2. **Buckwheat preparation:** - Thoroughly rinse and drain the raw buckwheat groats under cold running water.

3. **Combine the Ingredients:** - In a large mixing basin, blend together the ground cinnamon, unsweetened shredded coconut, chopped macadamia nuts, dried cranberries, and a little amount of salt (if desired).

4. **Add Sweetener and Oil:** - Pour olive oil and honey, or another sugar alternative, over the mixture. Make sure that every dry ingredient is uniformly covered by giving it a good stir.

5. **Transfer to a baking sheet:** Evenly spread the mixture over the baking sheet that has been ready.

6. **Bake:** Bake for 20 to 25 minutes, or until the granola is crisp and golden, in a preheated oven. To guarantee even browning, stir the granola every ten minutes.

7. **Cool and Store:**

- Let the granola cool on the baking sheet entirely. It will get crispier as it cools.

- After the granola cools, move it to a storage container that can seal tightly.

Estimated Preparation Time:

After baking and cooling, this recipe for Buckwheat Granola with Macadamia Nuts and Cranberries takes around 35 to 40 minutes.

Nutritional Value (about, per 1/4 cup serving):

There are 150–170 calories.

- 3–4 grams of protein

- 2–3 grams of fiber

- 100–150 mg of potassium and 50–70 mg of phosphorus

- Sodium: Changes according to salt addition

- Haddock and kale kedgeree:

Ingredients:

- Two haddock fillets, about 6 ounces each

- Two cups low-sodium vegetable broth - One cup long-grain white rice

- Two cups chopped kale (stems removed)

- One little onion, cut finely;

- Two minced garlic cloves

- One-tsp curry powder

- 1/4 teaspoon each of ground cumin,

- 1/4 teaspoon each of powdered coriander,

- 1/2 teaspoon of ground turmeric

- 1/4 cup rice or almond milk, or other low-potassium milk

- Two hard-boiled eggs, chopped and peeled;

- Two teaspoons of freshly chopped parsley

- To taste, add salt and pepper

- Use olive oil while cooking

Instructions:

1. **Get the haddock ready:** Sprinkle a little salt and pepper on the haddock fillets. A little bit of olive oil in a pan on a medium heat. Flake the haddock fillets with a fork by cooking them for approximately 3–4 minutes on each side. After the haddock is done, take it out of the skillet and reserve.

2. **Prepare the Rice:** Place the long-grain white rice and low-sodium vegetable broth in a different pot. Once it reaches a boil, lower the heat to a simmer, cover, and let the rice cook for 15 to 20 minutes, or until it is soft and the liquid has been absorbed.

3. **Sauté the Onion and Kale:** - If necessary, add a little extra olive oil to the same skillet that was used to cook the haddock. The minced garlic and finely diced onion should be sautéed until they are transparent and tender. Add the chopped kale and heat until it wilts, about 2 to 3 minutes more.

4. **Include milk and spices:**

- Add the ground coriander, cumin, turmeric, and curry powder and stir. To toast the spices, cook for one more minute.

- Add the low-potassium milk and whisk to get a sauce that is creamy.

5. **Merge and Arrange:**

- Add the cooked haddock, along with the greens and spicy sauce, to the skillet after flaking it. Mix the ingredients together gently.

- Add the cooked rice and stir until all the ingredients are thoroughly combined. To taste, add salt and pepper for seasoning.

6. Serve:

- Place the chopped hard-boiled eggs and fresh parsley on top of the plate containing the haddock and kale kedgeree.

Estimated Preparation Time:

Cooking time for this haddock and kale kedgeree dish is about 45 to 50 minutes.

Nutritional Value (about, per serving):

- 350 and 400 calories

- 30 to 35 grams of protein

- 4–6 grams of fiber

- 350–400 mg of potassium

- 250–300 mg of phosphorus

- Sodium: Changes according to salt addition

- Sip and Enjoy: Diabetic-Friendly Shakes and Smoothies

- Berry Concoction

- ¼ cup cranberry juice cocktail

- 1/3 cup firm silken tofu

- ½ cup frozen, unsweetened raspberries

- ½ cup frozen, unsweetened blueberries

- One tsp vanilla essence

Transfer the juice to a blender. Add the remaining components. Until extremely smooth, blend. Serve right away.

Nutritional Value

- portion size: one cup

- 188 calories

- 28 grams of carbohydrates

- 8 of grams protein

- 7 grams of dietary fiber

- 3 grams of fat

- Six milligrams sodium

- A total of 163 mg of potassium

- Thirty milligrams of phosphorus

- **Apple-Banana Smoothie**

- Half a banana, chopped into bits after peeling.

- Half a cup of yogurt

- ½ cup unsweetened applesauce

- 1/4 cup rice or almond milk

- 1 Teaspoon honey

- Two teaspoons of wheat bran or oats

In a blender, combine the banana, yogurt, applesauce, milk, and honey. Mix until homogeneous. Blend in oat bran until it thickens.

Nutritional Value

portion size: one cup

- 292 calories

- Grams of carbohydrates: 61

- Nine grams of protein

- 103 milligrams of sodium

- 609 milligrams of potassium

- 140 milligrams of phosphorus

- **Simple Milkless Shake**

- ½ C Pasteurized Egg Product in Liquid Form

- ½ C Frozen Whipped Topping Without Dairy

- Selective flavor: vanilla extract, lemon juice, or almond extract

- A quarter cup of berries, an apple, a banana, or two teaspoons of peanut butter

Nutritional Value

portion size: one cup

- 203 calories

- 19 g protein

- 195 mg of sodium

- 52 milligrams of potassium.

-1 milligrams of phosphorus

in addition to the minerals enhanced by peanut butter and taste

- **Smoothie with blueberries blast**

Ingredients:

- 1/2 cup of low-potassium frozen blueberries

- Half a cup of plain apple juice

- 1/2 cup of low-potassium yogurt, such as almond or Greek yogurt

- Half of a ripe banana

- 1/2 cup of optionally added ice cubes for thickness

- One tablespoon of honey, or sugar alternative (to taste)

Instructions:

1. **Assemble the ingredients:**

- Ensure that every component is prepared.

2. **Blend it all:**

- Place the frozen blueberries, ripe banana, low-potassium yogurt, unsweetened apple juice, and ice cubes (if using) in a blender.

- Add honey or a sugar substitute to taste if you'd like your smoothie to be sweeter.

3. **Puree until silky:**

- Process the mixture in a blender until the ingredients are smooth and creamy. You may adjust the thickness by adding a small amount extra apple juice if it's too thick.

4. **Taste and Modify:** Taste the smoothie and add extra honey, sugar substitute, or apple juice to modify the sweetness or thickness as necessary.

5. **Serve:** Fill a glass with the Blueberry Blast Smoothie and savor!

Estimated Preparation Time:

Making this Blueberry Blast Smoothie takes around five minutes.

Nutritional Value (approximately, for one serving):

- 150 and 200 calories

- 5 to 7 grams of protein

- 3–4 grams of fiber

- 150–200 milligrams of potassium

- 100–150 mg of phosphorus

- Sodium: Varies according on ingredients and salt addition.

- **Simple Protein Smoothie with Pineapples**

Ingredients:

- 1/2 cup fresh or canned pineapple pieces, without added sugar

- 1/2 cup of low-potassium yogurt, such as almond or Greek yogurt

- 1/2 cup rice or almond milk, or other low-potassium milk

- One scoop of protein powder low in potassium and phosphorus (see your dietician for appropriate selections)

- A half of a ripe banana, optional for extra creaminess

- 1/2 cup of optionally added ice cubes for thickness

- One tablespoon of honey, or sugar alternative (to taste)

Instructions:

1. **Get Your Ingredients Ready:** Make sure that every component is prepared.

2. **Mix together in the blender:** Place the unsweetened pineapple pieces, protein powder, low-potassium yogurt, low-potassium milk, and the ripe banana (if using) in a blender.

3. **Add sugar to taste:** You may taste and add honey or a sugar alternative if you like your smoothie sweeter.

4. **For thickness, add ice:** To get a more dense consistency, add ice cubes.

5. **Puree until silky:** Process the mixture in a blender until the ingredients are smooth and creamy. If necessary, adjust the thickness by adding extra milk or ice.

6. **Taste and Modify:** After tasting your pineapple protein smoothie, taste it and adjust the sweetness, thickness, and other ingredients to your liking.

6. **Serve:** Fill a glass with your Easy Pineapple Protein Smoothie and enjoy the delicious tropical flavor!

Estimated Preparation Time:

Making this simple pineapple protein smoothie should take five to seven minutes.

Nutritional Value (approximately, for one serving):

- 250 and 300 calories

- 15–20 grams of protein

- 2–3 grams of fiber

- 250–300 milligrams of potassium

- 100–150 mg of phosphorus

- Sodium: Varies according on ingredients and salt addition.

- Fruity Drink

Ingredients:

- 1/2 cup of low-potassium frozen mixed berries

- Half of a ripe banana

- 1/2 cup of low-potassium yogurt, such as almond or Greek yogurt

- 1/2 cup rice or almond milk, or other low-potassium milk

- 1/2 cup of optionally added ice cubes for thickness

- One tablespoon of honey, or sugar alternative (to taste)

Instructions:

1. **Get Your Ingredients Ready:** Ensure that every component is prepared.

2. **Combine the Fruits:** Place the ripe banana and frozen mixed berries in a blender.

3. **Add the sweetener and dairy:** Fill the blender with the low-potassium milk and yogurt. Add honey or a sugar alternative to taste if you want your smoothie to be sweeter.

4. **Use Ice to Thicken:** You may add ice cubes to the blender to achieve a thicker thickness.

5. **Puree until silky:** Process all the ingredients in a blender until a smooth, creamy consistency is achieved for your fruit smoothie. You can add additional milk or ice as needed to change the thickness.

6. **Taste and Modify:** After tasting the smoothie, adjust the sweetness, thickness, and other ingredients to your liking.

6. **Serve:** Fill a glass with your delectable Fruity Smoothie and enjoy all that fruit!

Estimated Preparation Time:

It takes around five to seven minutes to create this fruity smoothie.

Nutritional Value (approximately, for one serving):

- 200 and 250 calories

- 7–10 grams of protein

- 3–4 grams of fiber

- 200–250 milligrams of potassium

- 100–150 mg of phosphorus

- Sodium: Varies according on ingredients and salt addition.

- **Protein Smoothie with Mixed Berries**

Ingredients:

- 1/2 cup of low-potassium frozen mixed berries

- 1/2 cup of low-potassium yogurt, such as almond or Greek yogurt

- 1/2 cup rice or almond milk, or other low-potassium milk

- One scoop of protein powder low in potassium and phosphorus (see your dietician for appropriate selections)

- A half of a ripe banana, optional for extra creaminess

- 1/2 cup of optionally added ice cubes for thickness

- One tablespoon of honey, or sugar alternative (to taste)

Instructions:

1. **Assemble the ingredients:** Make sure that every component is prepared.

2. **Mix together in the blender:** Place the frozen mixed berries, protein powder, low-potassium yogurt, low-potassium milk, and the ripe banana (if using) into a blender.

3. **Add sugar to taste:** You may taste and add honey or a sugar alternative if you like your smoothie sweeter.

4. **For thickness, add ice:** To get a more dense consistency, add ice cubes.

5. **Puree until silky:** Process the mixture in a blender until the ingredients are smooth and creamy. If necessary, adjust the thickness by adding extra milk or ice.

6. **Taste and Modify:** Taste your Mixed Berry Protein Smoothie and make any necessary adjustments to the sweetness, thickness, or other ingredients.

Fill a glass with your energizing Mixed Berry Protein Smoothie and have a nutritious and filling delight!

Estimated Preparation Time:

Making this Mixed Berry Protein Smoothie will take around five to seven minutes.

Nutritional Value (approximately, for one serving):

- 250 and 300 calories

- 15–20 grams of protein

- 2–3 grams of fiber

- 250–300 milligrams of potassium

- 100–150 mg of phosphorus

- Sodium: Varies according on ingredients and salt addition.

- **High-Protein Peach Smoothie**

Ingredients:

- One cup of low-potassium frozen peaches

- 1/2 cup of low-potassium yogurt, such as almond or Greek yogurt

- 1/2 cup rice or almond milk, or other low-potassium milk

- One scoop of protein powder low in potassium and phosphorus (see your dietician for appropriate selections)

- 1/2 cup of optionally added ice cubes for thickness

- One tablespoon of honey, or sugar alternative (to taste)

Instructions:

1. **Get Your Ingredients Ready**: Verify that every ingredient is prepared.

2. **Mix together in the blender:** Place the frozen peaches, protein powder, low-potassium yogurt, low-potassium milk, and honey (or sugar replacement) in a blender.

3. **Modify Thickness:** Add ice cubes if you like a thicker consistency.

4. **Puree until silky:** Process all the ingredients in your blender until a smooth and creamy peach high-protein smoothie is achieved. If necessary, adjust the thickness by adding extra milk or ice.

5. **Taste and Modify:** After tasting your smoothie, adjust the sweetness, thickness, and other ingredients to your preferred levels.

Transfer your Peach High-Protein Smoothie into a glass and savor this tasty and nourishing beverage!

Estimated Preparation Time:

Making this Peach High-Protein Smoothie will take about five to seven minutes.

Nutritional Value (approximately, for one serving):

- 250 and 300 calories

- 15–20 grams of protein

- 2–3 grams of fiber

- 200–250 milligrams of potassium

- 100–150 mg of phosphorus

- Sodium: Varies according on ingredients and salt addition.

Smoothie with Strawberry High-Protein

Ingredients:

- One cup of frozen potassium-low strawberries

- 1/2 cup of low-potassium yogurt, such as almond or Greek yogurt

- 1/2 cup rice or almond milk, or other low-potassium milk

- One scoop of protein powder low in potassium and phosphorus (see your dietician for appropriate selections)

- 1/2 cup of optionally added ice cubes for thickness

- One tablespoon of honey, or sugar alternative (to taste)

Instructions:

1. **Assemble the ingredients:** Make sure that every component is prepared.

2. **Mix together in the blender:** Combine the protein powder, low-potassium yogurt, low-potassium milk, frozen strawberries, and honey (or sugar replacement) in a blender.

3. **Modify Thickness:** Add ice cubes if you like a thicker consistency.

4. **Puree until silky:** Process all ingredients in a blender until a smooth and creamy strawberry high-protein smoothie is achieved. If necessary, adjust the thickness by adding extra milk or ice.

5. **Taste and Modify:** After tasting your smoothie, adjust the sweetness, thickness, and other ingredients to your preferred levels.

Fill a glass with your Strawberry High-Protein Smoothie and enjoy this tasty and nourishing treat!

Estimated Preparation Time:

Making this Strawberry High-Protein Smoothie will take about five to seven minutes.

Nutritional Value (approximately, for one serving):

- 250 and 300 calories

- 15–20 grams of protein

- 2–3 grams of fiber

- 200–250 milligrams of potassium

- 100–150 mg of phosphorus

- Sodium: Varies according on ingredients and salt addition.

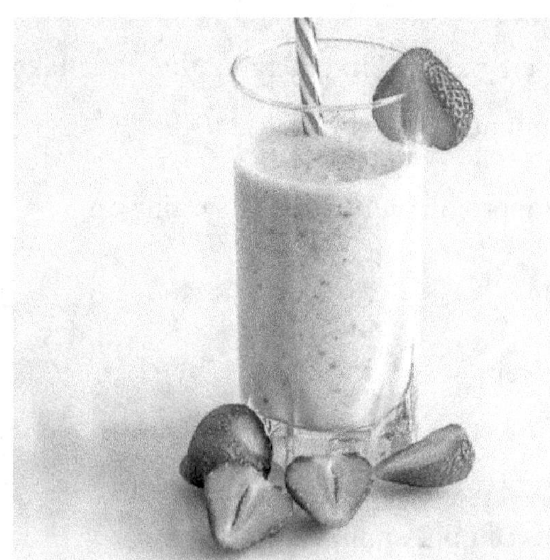

CHAPTER FOUR

Lunchtime Wonders

- A Harmony of Tastes: Salads and Wraps

- Hawaiian Chicken Salad Sandwich

Ingredients:

For the Chicken Salad:

- Two cups of cooked, low-potassium chicken breast, shredded or cubed

- 1/2 cup plain Greek yogurt with low potassium

- 1/4 cup chopped low-potassium pineapple, either fresh or canned.

- 1/4 cup finely chopped celery

- 2 teaspoons finely chopped red onion

- One tablespoon of chopped unsalted macadamia nuts (optional)

- One-half tsp curry powder

- To taste, add salt and pepper.

For the Sandwich:

- Four slices of low-sodium, kidney-friendly bread

- Leaf lettuce

- Slices of tomato (optional)

- Leaves of spinach or Swiss chard (optional)

Instructions:

1. **Get the chicken salad ready by:**

- Put the cooked chicken, diced pineapple, finely chopped celery, red onion, and unsalted macadamia nuts (if using) in a mixing bowl. Do not stir. Blend well.

- Add the curry powder and taste and adjust with salt and pepper. Mix everything up thoroughly by stirring.

2. **Put the Sandwich Together:**

- Top one piece of bread that is good for your kidneys with a lettuce leaf.

- Evenly distribute a large amount of the Hawaiian chicken salad over the lettuce.

- For more taste and freshness, feel free to add spinach leaves, tomato slices, or Swiss chard.

- To make a sandwich, place another slice of bread on top.

3.**Serve:** After cutting the sandwich in half, serve it. You may serve it with your preferred side dish or a side salad that is low in potassium.

Estimated Preparation Time:

Making this Hawaiian Chicken Salad Sandwich, assuming you have cooked chicken on hand, should take around 15 to 20 minutes.

Nutritional Value (about, per sandwich):

- Between 350 and 400 calories

- 30 to 35 grams of protein

- 3–4 grams of fiber

- 250–300 milligrams of potassium

- 200–250 mg of phosphorus

- 150–200 milligrams of sodium

- Italian Chicken Salad

Ingredients:

For the Chicken Salad:

- Two cups of cooked, low-potassium chicken breast, shredded or cubed

- 1/4 cup plain Greek yogurt with low potassium

- 1/4 cup mayonnaise with reduced potassium

- 1/4 cup finely chopped sun-dried tomatoes (with oil; remove excess)

- Two tablespoons of low-phosphorus grated Parmesan cheese

- 1 tablespoon finely chopped fresh basil

- Half a teaspoon of oregano, dry

- To taste, add salt and pepper.

For the Salad:

- Four cups of mixed greens, such as arugula, spinach, and lettuce

- One cup of chopped cherry tomatoes

- Half a cucumber, cut

- 1/4 finely sliced red onion

- 1/4 cup low-sodium black olives, if desired

Instructions:

1. Chicken salad preparation:

- Place the cooked chicken, chopped sun-dried tomatoes, low-potassium Greek yogurt, low-potassium mayonnaise, grated Parmesan cheese, fresh basil, dried oregano, and salt and pepper to taste in a mixing dish. Blend well.

2. Put the Salad Together:

- Mix the greens and place them in a big serving basin.

- Add the cucumber slices, black olives (if using), cherry tomato halves, and thinly sliced red onion.

3. Serve:

- Spoon the mixed greens and vegetables onto the bed of Italian chicken salad.

- If wanted, garnish with more fresh basil and Parmesan cheese.

- Before serving, toss the salad ingredients together or top with the chicken salad.

Estimated Preparation Time:

With cooked chicken on hand, this Italian Chicken Salad may be made in about 15 to 20 minutes.

Nutritional Value (about, per serving):

- Between 350 and 400 calories

- 30 to 35 grams of protein

- 5–6 grams of fiber

- 350–400 mg of potassium

- 200–250 mg of phosphorus

Salinity: 200–250 mg

- **Salad with Fruited Curry Chicken**

Ingredients:

For the Chicken Salad:

- Two cups of cooked, low-potassium chicken breast, shredded or cubed

- 1/4 cup plain Greek yogurt with low potassium

- 1/4 cup mayonnaise with reduced potassium

- 1/4 cup of raisins or dried cranberries

- Two tablespoons of finely chopped, low-phosphorus almonds

- One tablespoon of honey, or sugar alternative (to taste)

- One-tsp curry powder

- To taste, add salt and pepper.

For the Salad:

- Four cups of mixed greens, such as arugula, spinach, and lettuce

- Half a chopped red apple (poor in potassium)

- Half a cup of seedless, low-potassium grapes

- 1/4 finely sliced red onion

Instructions:

1. **Chicken salad preparation:**

- Place the cooked chicken, low-potassium Greek yogurt, low-potassium mayonnaise, sliced almonds, dried cranberries or raisins, curry powder, honey (or sugar alternative), and salt and pepper to taste in a mixing bowl. Blend well.

2. **Put the Salad Together:**

- Mix the greens and place them in a big serving basin.

- Add the thinly sliced red onion, chopped red apple, and half seedless grapes.

- Place a scoop of the fruit-and-curry chicken salad on top of the fruit-and-greens bed.

- Make sure the chicken salad melds with the fruits and greens for a tasty and reviving blend by tossing the salad well before serving.

Estimated Preparation Time:

If you have cooked chicken on hand, this Fruited Curry Chicken Salad should only take 15 to 20 minutes to create.

Nutritional Value (about, per serving):

- 350 and 400 calories

- 30 to 35 grams of protein

- 4–5 grams of fiber

- 250–300 milligrams of potassium

- 200–250 mg of phosphorus

- 150–200 milligrams of sodium

- **Pineapple-Basil Lime Salad**

Ingredients:

- Two cups of fresh, chopped pineapple (low in potassium)

- 1/4 cup finely sliced fresh basil leaves

- One tablespoon of lime juice, fresh

- One tablespoon of honey, or sugar alternative (to taste)

- Scent of one lime

- To taste, freshly ground black pepper

- Optional fresh mint leaves as a garnish

Instructions:

1. **Get the pineapple ready:**

- Chop the fresh pineapple into small pieces using a knife. When using canned pineapple, make sure it has been thoroughly drained and select pineapple that is packaged in juice rather than syrup.

2. **Prepare the Garnish:** Place the fresh lime juice, lime zest, and honey (or sugar alternative) in a small bowl. Blend well.

3. **Blend the Ingredients:** Gently mix the thinly cut basil leaves and cubed pineapple in a serving basin.

4. **Dress It Up:** Pour the lime dressing over the combination of pineapple and basil. Gently toss to evenly coat the fruit and herbs.

5. **Garnish and Season:** To taste, add freshly ground black pepper to the salad. Garnish with fresh mint leaves for an added taste boost, if preferred.

6. **Serve:** To achieve the finest flavor, let the ingredients of the basil-lime pineapple salad meld together in the refrigerator for approximately half an hour.

Estimated Preparation Time:

Making this Basil-Lime Pineapple Salad takes fifteen to twenty minutes.

Nutritional Value (about, per serving):

- Energy content: 80–100 calories

- 2–3 grams of fiber

- 150–200 milligrams of potassium

- Potassium: 10–20 mg

- Sodium: Changes according to salt addition

- **Salad with Chicken Apple Crunch.**

Ingredients:

For the Salad:

- Two cups of cooked, low-potassium chicken breast, shredded or cubed

- Two cups of mixed greens, such as arugula, spinach, and lettuce

- One chopped red apple (low in potassium)

- 1/4 cup finely chopped celery

- 1/4 cup chopped, low-phosphorus walnuts

- 1/4 cup finely chopped red onion

For the Dressing:

– Two tablespoons low-sodium mayo

- Two tablespoons of plain Greek yogurt with low potassium

- One tablespoon of honey, or sugar alternative (to taste)

- One tsp of apple cider vinegar

- To taste, add salt and pepper.

Instructions:

1. **Get the salad ready:** Place the cooked chicken, mixed greens, diced apple, chopped walnuts, finely chopped celery, and thinly sliced red onion in a large salad dish.

2. **Prepare the Garnish:** Combine the low-potassium Greek yogurt, low-potassium mayonnaise, apple cider vinegar, honey (or sugar alternative), and salt and pepper to taste in a separate bowl.

3. **Mix Salad and Dressing Together:** Drizzle the salad with the dressing, tossing gently to cover every component equally.

4. Cool and Present: To allow the flavors to mingle, chill the chicken apple crunch salad for 15 to 20 minutes.

Estimated Preparation Time:

Making this Chicken Apple Crunch Salad, assuming you have cooked chicken on hand, should take around 15 to 20 minutes.

Nutritional Value (about, per serving):

- 350 and 400 calories

- 30 to 35 grams of protein

- 4–5 grams of fiber

- 300–350 milligrams of potassium

- 100–150 mg of phosphorus

- 150–200 milligrams of sodium

- **Crispy Salad of Couscous**

Ingredients:

For the Salad:

- One cup of potassium-low whole wheat couscous

- 1 1/2 cups water or low-sodium vegetable broth

- 1/4 cup chopped cucumber

- 1/4 cup chopped red bell pepper

- 1/4 cup coarsely chopped red onion

- 1/4 cup finely chopped celery

- 1/4 cup of halved cherry tomatoes

- 1/4 cup finely chopped fresh parsley

- 1/4 cup low-potassium canned chickpeas, washed and drained

- 1/4 cup of low-phosphorus unsalted sunflower seeds

For the Dressing:

- Two tsp olive oil

- Two tsp freshly squeezed lemon juice

- One teaspoon of honey, or sugar alternative (to taste)

- To taste, add salt and pepper.

Instructions:

1. **Get the couscous ready:**

- Bring water or low-sodium vegetable broth to a boil in a medium pot. Add the whole wheat couscous and stir.

- After turning off the heat and covering, wait five minutes or so for the couscous to absorb the liquid. Using a fork, fluff and allow to cool.

2. **Prepare the Garnish:** Combine the olive oil, lemon juice (fresh or preserved), honey (or sugar alternative), salt, and pepper in a small bowl. Put away.

3. **Put the Salad Together:** Place the cooked and cooled couscous, diced cucumber, red bell pepper, celery, cherry tomatoes, finely sliced red onion, fresh parsley, chickpeas, and sunflower seeds in a large salad dish.

4. **Add the Garnish:** Pour the dressing over the salad and gently toss to ensure that all of the items are coated.

5. **Chill and Serve:** To enable the flavors to mingle, chill the Crunchy Couscous Salad for fifteen to twenty minutes before serving.

Estimated Preparation Time:

Allowing the couscous to cool down will add another twenty to twenty-five minutes to the preparation time of this crunchy couscous salad.

Nutritional Value (about, per serving):

- Between 300 and 350 calories

- 9–11 grams of protein

- 5–6 grams of fiber

- 200–250 milligrams of potassium

- 100–150 mg of phosphorus

- 100–150 mg of sodium

- Liquid Remedies: Low-Sodium Soups

- Chicken Soup with Low Sodium

Ingredients:

- Two cooked, thinly sliced, low-sodium boneless, skinless chicken breasts

- A tsp of olive oil

- 1/2 cup finely chopped onions

- 1/2 cup finely chopped celery

- 1/2 cup finely sliced carrots

- Two minced garlic cloves

- Eight cups chicken broth reduced in sodium

- One cup of drained, low-sodium canned corn (optional; poor in potassium)

- One cup of finely chopped green beans

- 1/2 cup elbows or little shells pasta, low in salt

- One bay leaf

- One-half tsp dried thyme

- An alternative to salt (optional, to taste)

- To taste, freshly ground black pepper

- Chopped fresh parsley, optional as a garnish

Instructions:

1. **Let the chicken cook and shred.**

- Heat the olive oil in a big saucepan over medium heat. Stir in the carrots, celery, and onion. Sauté them for five minutes or until they start to get tender.

- Add the minced garlic and continue cooking for an additional minute.

2. **Simmer after adding broth:**

- Add the shredded chicken, spaghetti, green beans, canned corn (if using), bay leaf, and dried thyme to the low-sodium chicken broth.

- After bringing the soup to a boil, lower the heat, and simmer it until the noodles and veggies are soft, about 10 to 15 minutes

3. **Season to Taste:** Use freshly ground black pepper and a salt alternative to season the soup as needed. The salt replacement can be rather salty, so use caution while using it. Start with a tiny quantity and titrate to your preference.

Remember to take out the bay leaf from the soup before serving. Spoon into bowls the Low Sodium Chicken Soup. Add some freshly chopped parsley as a garnish if you want a little pop of freshness.

Estimated Preparation Time:

When all of the chicken is cooked and shredded, this low-sodium chicken soup should be ready in 30 to 40 minutes.

Nutritional Value (about, per serving):

- 150 and 200 calories

- 15–20 grams of protein

- 3–4 grams of fiber

- 150–200 milligrams of potassium

- 100–150 mg of phosphorus

- Sodium: 100–150 mg (sodium excluded)

- **Roasted Chicken Noodle with Lower Sodium**

Ingredients:

- Two cooked, thinly sliced, low-sodium boneless, skinless chicken breasts

- A tsp of olive oil

- 1/2 cup finely chopped onions

- 1/2 cup finely chopped celery

- 1/2 cup finely sliced carrots

- Two minced garlic cloves

- Eight cups chicken broth reduced in sodium

- One cup of drained, low-sodium canned corn (optional; poor in potassium)

- One cup of finely chopped green beans

- 1/2 cup elbows or little shells pasta, low in salt

- One bay leaf

- One-half tsp dried thyme

- An alternative to salt (optional, to taste)

- To taste, freshly ground black pepper

- Chopped fresh parsley, optional as a garnish

Instructions:

1. **Let the chicken cook and shred.**

- Heat the olive oil in a big saucepan over medium heat. Stir in the carrots, celery, and onion. Sauté them for five minutes or until they start to get tender.

- Add the minced garlic and continue cooking for an additional minute.

2. **Simmer after adding broth:**

- Add the shredded chicken, spaghetti, green beans, canned corn (if using), bay leaf, and dried thyme to the low-sodium chicken broth.

- After bringing the soup to a boil, lower the heat, and simmer it until the noodles and veggies are soft, about 10 to 15 minutes.

3. **Season to Taste:** Use freshly ground black pepper and a salt alternative to season the soup as needed. The salt replacement can be rather salty, so use caution while using it. Start with a tiny quantity and titrate to your preference.

Spoon the Roasted Chicken Noodle Soup with Reduced Sodium into individual bowls. Add some freshly chopped parsley as a garnish if you want a little pop of freshness.

Estimated Preparation Time:

The roasting and shredding of the chicken will take around 30 to 40 minutes for this reduced-sodium roasted chicken noodle soup to come together.

Nutritional Value (about, per serving):

- 150 and 200 calories

- 15–20 grams of protein

- 3–4 grams of fiber

- 150–200 milligrams of potassium

- 100–150 mg of phosphorus

- Sodium: 100–150 mg (sodium excluded)

- **Tomato Bisque with Chunks**

Ingredients:

- Two tsp olive oil

- 1/2 cup finely chopped onions

- 1/2 cup finely chopped celery

- 1/2 cup finely sliced carrots

- Two minced garlic cloves

- One 28-ounce container of chopped tomatoes with minimal sodium

- 1/2 cup vegetarian broth reduced in sodium

- One-half tsp dried basil

- Half a teaspoon of oregano, dry

- One-half tsp dried thyme

- An alternative to salt (optional, to taste)

- To taste, freshly ground black pepper

- Fresh basil leaves, optional as a garnish

Instructions:

1. **Cook the Veggies**: Heat the olive oil in a big saucepan over medium heat. Stir in the carrots, celery, and onion. Sauté the veggies for five to seven minutes, or until they begin to soften.

2. **Add the seasonings and tomatoes:**

- Add the minced garlic and continue cooking for an additional minute.

- Add the dried basil, dried oregano, and dried thyme, along with the low-sodium diced tomatoes and their juice and low-sodium vegetable broth.

3. Cook the Soup: After bringing the mixture to a boil, turn down the heat. Simmer for fifteen to twenty minutes, stirring once and again.

4. Mix up the Soup: Blend the soup with an immersion blender or move it to a countertop blender in batches. Blend until you have the consistency you want—straight or slightly chunky—that is.

5. Use freshly ground black pepper and a salt alternative to season the soup as needed. Start with a tiny quantity and titrate to your preference.

6. Garnish and Serve: Pour dishes with the chunky tomato bisque. Add some fresh basil leaves as a garnish if you want to add some color and freshness.

Estimated Preparation Time:

The preparation of this chunky tomato bisque should take thirty to forty minutes.

Nutritional Value (about, per serving):

- 80–100 calories

- 2–3 grams of protein

- 3–4 grams of fiber

- 250–300 milligrams of potassium

- Potassium: 30–40 mg

- 100–150 mg of sodium

- **Light in Sous Vide Sodium Minestrone**

Ingredients:

- A tsp of olive oil

- 1/2 cup finely chopped onions

- 1/2 cup finely chopped celery

- 1/2 cup finely sliced carrots

- Two minced garlic cloves

– 4 cups vegetable broth with minimal sodium

- One 14-ounce container of chopped tomatoes with minimal sodium

- One cup washed and drained low-sodium kidney beans

- 1/2 cup finely chopped low-sodium green beans

- 1/2 cup sliced low-sodium zucchini

- 1/2 cup elbows or little shells pasta, low in salt

– One tsp. dried basil

- One teaspoon of oregano, dried

- An alternative to salt (optional, to taste)

- To taste, freshly ground black pepper

- Chopped fresh parsley, optional as a garnish

- Grated Parmesan cheese (low-phosphorus optional)

Instructions:

1. **Cook the Veggies:** Heat the olive oil in a big saucepan over medium heat. Stir in the carrots, celery, and onion. When the veggies start to soften, sauté them for five to seven minutes.

2. **Add the tomatoes and broth.**

- Add the minced garlic and continue cooking for an additional minute.

- Add the low-sodium chopped tomatoes (with their juice) and pour in the low-sodium vegetable broth.

3. **Add the ingredients and simmer:**

- Once the mixture reaches a boil, turn down the heat. Simmer it for ten to fifteen minutes.

- Add the dried oregano and basil, as well as the low-sodium kidney beans, low-sodium green beans, low-sodium zucchini, and low-sodium pasta. Simmer the noodles and veggies until they are cooked.

4. **Season to Taste**: Use freshly ground black pepper and a salt alternative to season the soup as needed. Start with a tiny quantity and titrate to your preference. Spoon Sodium Minestrone Soup Light into individual dishes. Add some freshly chopped parsley and grated Parmesan cheese, if you can handle it because it's low in phosphorus, as garnish.

Estimated Preparation Time:

The preparation of this Light in Sodium Minestrone Soup should take about 30 to 40 minutes.

Nutritional Value (about, per serving):

- 100 and 150 calories

- 4–5 grams of protein

- 4–5 grams of fiber

- 200–250 milligrams of potassium

- Cadmium: 50–60 mg

- Sodium: 100–150 mg (without added salt)

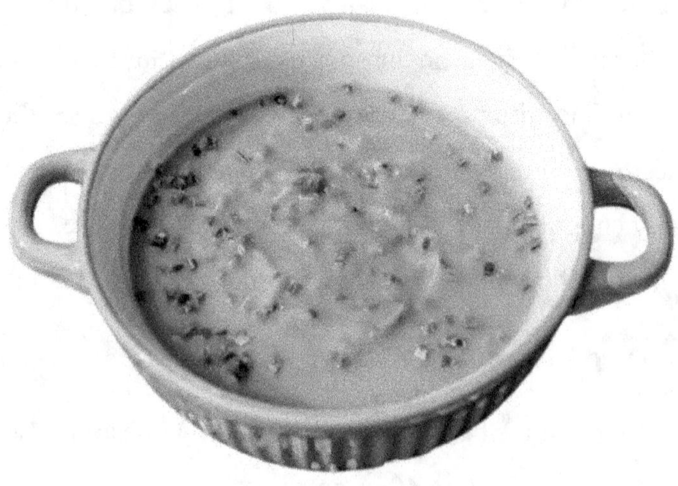

CHAPTER FIVE

Supper Treats: A Kidney-Friendly Feast

- Make Main Courses That Are Kidney-Friendly.

- Fish baked over rice or pasta

Ingredients:

- Four white fish fillets, skinless and boneless (such as cod, haddock, or tilapia)

- One cup of long-grain white rice, or your preferred kidney-friendly pasta

- Two cups low-sodium vegetable or chicken broth

- One finely sliced lemon

- Two tsp olive oil

- One teaspoon of oregano, dried

- A teaspoon of thyme, dried

- To taste, add salt and pepper.

- Fresh parsley chopped for a garnish

Instructions:

About the Pasta or Rice:

1. Turn the oven on to 375°F, or 190°C.

2. Bring the low-sodium chicken or vegetable broth to a boil in a medium-sized pot.

3. When the broth reaches a rolling boil, add the rice (or kidney-friendly pasta), cover, lower the heat, and simmer the food until it is soft, following the cooking instructions on the rice or pasta box. Take it off the stove and cover it for a few minutes before using a fork to fluff it up.

For the Fish Bake:

1. Prepare the fish while the rice (or pasta) is cooking. Arrange the fish fillets onto a parchment paper-lined baking sheet.

2. Season the fish fillets with salt, pepper, dried thyme, and dried oregano by drizzling them with olive oil. Rub the fish with the spice, gently.

3. Place the slices of lemon on top of the fish fillets.

4. Fish should be baked in a preheated oven for 15 to 20 minutes, or until a fork can easily pierce it and the sides begin to softly brown.

To Serve

1. Spoon the cooked pasta or rice onto four dishes.

2. Top each plate of rice (or spaghetti) with a roasted fish fillet.

3. Add some fresh parsley as a garnish for color and taste.

4. Depending on your dietary preferences, serve your kidney-friendly Baked Fish with Rice (or Pasta) with a fresh salad or steamed veggies.

- Corn on the cob with flank steak

Ingredients:

- One-pound steak on the flank

- Four freshly picked corn kernels

- A tsp of olive oil

- One teaspoon powdered garlic

- One tsp of paprika

- To taste, add salt and pepper.

- Fresh parsley chopped for a garnish

Instructions:

For the Flank Steak:

1. Set your grill's temperature to medium-high.

2. To make a marinade, combine the olive oil, paprika, garlic powder, salt, and pepper in a small bowl.

3. Make sure the flank steak is equally covered on both sides by brushing it with the marinade.

4. For medium-rare, cook the marinated flank steak on the grill for three to four minutes on each side. You may modify the cooking time according to the doneness you want.

5. After the steak is cooked to your preference, take it from the grill and give it some time to rest before slicing it into thin pieces.

For the Cob of Corn:

1. Prepare the corn on the cob while the steak is resting.

2. Pour water into a big saucepan and heat it until it boils.

3. When the water is boiling, add the corn ears and simmer for 7 to 8 minutes, or until the corn is soft.

4. After draining, let the corn to cool somewhat.

To Serve:

1. Thinly slice the flank steak that has been grilled.

2. Present the corn on the cob with the steak slices on the side.

3. Add some chopped fresh parsley as a garnish to the steak to improve appearance and flavor.

4. Serve this meal, if desired, with a kidney-friendly sauce or a squeeze of fresh lemon for added flavor.

- Stir-fry mélange of beef and vegetables

Ingredients:

- One pound of thinly sliced lean protein, such as turkey, chicken, or pork

- Two cups of carefully selected, sliced or diced kidney-friendly vegetables (such as bell peppers, broccoli, carrots, zucchini, or green beans).

- A spoonful of soy sauce with reduced sodium

- One tsp olive oil

- One minced garlic clove

- One tsp finely chopped ginger

- To taste, add salt and pepper.

- Finely chopped green onions, optional as a garnish

Instructions:

To make the stir-fry:

1. A big wok or pan should be heated to medium-high heat.

2. To the heated pan, add the olive oil.

3. Stir-fry the protein slices after adding them until they are fully cooked and no longer pink. It will take around four to six minutes, according on the kind of protein you use. The cooked protein should be taken out of the pan and placed aside.

4. Add the ginger and garlic, minced, to the same pan. Sauté until aromatic, approximately 30 seconds.

5. Fill the skillet with your preferred kidney-friendly veggies. Stir-fry for three to five minutes, or until they are crisp-tender.

6. Add the cooked protein and veggies back to the pan.

7. Pour the reduced-sodium soy sauce onto the meat and veggies. Mix well and cook for a further two minutes.

8. To taste, add salt and pepper for seasoning.

To Serve:

1. Spoon the meat and veggie mixture onto individual serving dishes.

2. If desired, add chopped green onions as a garnish for visual appeal and taste.

3. Depending on your dietary requirements, serve your kidney-friendly Stir Fry Meat and Vegetable Medley hot with steamed white rice or another kidney-friendly grain of your choosing.

- Salad of cabbage

Ingredients:

- Four cups of finely chopped green cabbage

– 1 cup finely sliced red cabbage

- One grated carrot

- 1/4 cup coarsely chopped red onion

- Two tablespoons of low-sodium vinegar, like white wine or apple cider vinegar

- A tsp of olive oil

- One teaspoon honey, or your preferred kidney-friendly sweetener

- To taste, add salt and pepper.

- Freshly chopped cilantro or parsley (optional)

Instructions:

1. Grated carrot, finely chopped red onion, red cabbage, and thinly sliced green cabbage should all be combined in a big mixing dish.

2. Make the dressing in a separate small bowl. Mix the olive oil, low-sodium vinegar, salt, pepper, honey (or other sweetener that is good for your kidneys), and honey. To suit your tastes, adjust the spice and sweetness.

3. Over the cabbage and vegetable combination, drizzle the dressing.

4. To make sure the dressing covers the cabbage and veggies equally, toss the ingredients well.

5. To let the flavors mingle, cover the bowl with plastic wrap and chill it in the refrigerator for at least half an hour. For even more taste, you may refrigerate it for a few hours.

6. If preferred, add some chopped fresh parsley or cilantro to the cabbage salad before serving.

7. Present the salad as a crisp and light entrée on its own, or as a cool side to go with your main course.

- **Eggplant kasha**

Ingredients:

- 1-cup kasha made from buckwheat

- two cups of water

- One chopped medium-sized eggplant

- One onion, diced finely

- Two minced garlic cloves

- Two tsp olive oil

- One 14-ounce can of chopped tomatoes without added salt

– One tsp. dried basil

- One teaspoon of oregano, dried

- To taste, add salt and pepper.

- Fresh parsley chopped (optional) as a garnish

Instructions:

For the Kasha:

1. Heat the water and buckwheat kasha in a medium pot. After bringing it to a boil, lower the heat to a simmer, cover it, and cook for ten to twelve minutes, or until the kasha is soft and the water has been absorbed. Using a fork, fluff and set aside.

For the Eggplant:

1. As the kasha cooks, get the eggplant ready. Transfer the chopped eggplant to a sieve and lightly season with salt. Give it a good fifteen minutes to sit. This aids in removing too much moisture.

2. Rinse the eggplant under cold water and blot dry with a fresh kitchen towel after 15 minutes.

3. Heat the olive oil in a big skillet over medium heat.

4. When the onion is transparent, add it and sauté it for three to four minutes.

5. When the garlic is aromatic, add the minced garlic and sauté for an additional 30 seconds.

6. Add the chopped eggplant and sauté it for 5-7 minutes, until it becomes soft and starts to color.

7. Add the dried oregano and basil, along with the can of chopped tomatoes (salted but not added). To taste, add salt and pepper for seasoning. Give everything a good stir, then boil it for five to seven minutes to let the flavors mingle.

To Serve:

1. The cooked buckwheat kasha can be served in bowls or on plates.

2. Arrange the eggplant and tomato mixture on top of the kasha.

3. If desired, garnish with freshly chopped parsley.

4. Present your nutritious and filling dish, rich in taste and texture, Eggplant Kasha, which is suitable for kidneys.

- Kare-kare (peanut stew) with vegetables

Ingredients:

- Two cups of sliced, round eggplant

- Two cups of green beans, sliced into 2-inch segments

- Two cups sliced butternut or calabaza squash

- One cup of string beans, optional, chopped into 2-inch pieces

- 1 cup sliced bok choy or Chinese cabbage

- 1/2 cup of unsweetened, unsalted peanut butter

- Chop one tiny onion.

- Two minced garlic cloves

– Two tsp of frying oil

- Four cups low-sodium vegetable broth

- 1/4 cup of optional shrimp paste (bagoong) for serving

- To taste, add salt and pepper.

Instructions:

1. Heat the cooking oil in a big saucepan over medium heat.

2. After the chopped onion has become transparent, add the minced garlic and continue to sauté. Saute for a further minute or until aromatic.

3. After adding the peanut butter, stir it in and let it melt slightly for a few minutes.

4. To get a smooth peanut sauce, add the vegetable broth gradually while stirring continuously. Heat the mixture until it simmers gently.

5. Put the squash, green beans, eggplant, and, if using, string beans into the saucepan. Simmer and simmer for 8 to 10 minutes, or until the veggies are mushy but not too so.

6. Add the chopped Chinese cabbage or bok choy to the saucepan. Simmer for a further two to three minutes, or until it wilts.

7. Add salt and pepper to taste and adjust the seasoning of the stew accordingly.

To Serve:

1. Spoon into dishes the Vegetable Kare-Kare.

2. For those who like the traditional condiment, serve it with a side of shrimp paste (bagoong) (optional).

3. Savor a full and flavorful lunch of kidney-friendly vegetable kare-kare while it's hot.

- **Learn About Vegetables and Sides In Kidney Cuisine**

- Almonds and cherries baked into apples

Ingredients:

- Four apples (choose a potassium-free type, like Granny Smith).

- 1/2 cup low-potassium, unsweetened dried cherries

- 1/4 cup of low-phosphorus chopped almonds

- 1/4 cup brown sugar replacement, adjusted for flavor

- Half a teaspoon of cinnamon, ground

- 1/4 teaspoon of nutmeg, ground

- One tablespoon of margarine or unsalted butter

Instructions:

1. **Warm up the oven:** Set the oven temperature to 175°C, or 350°F.

2. **Get the apples ready:** Clean and core the apples, taking out the seeds and making a little well to contain the filling in the middle. Don't cut off the apple's bottom.

3. **Get the Filling Ready:** Combine the chopped almonds, ground nutmeg, ground cinnamon, brown sugar replacement, and dried cherries in a mixing dish. Well combine the components.

4. **Load up the apples:** Carefully place the cherry and almond filling into each apple, making sure it fits snugly inside the well you made.

5. **Put in the butter:** To enhance taste and moisture, top each filled apple with a little dollop of unsalted butter or margarine.

6. **Bake:** The filled apples should be arranged in a baking dish. You may avoid sticking or burning by adding a small amount of water to the dish's bottom. Fold the foil over the dish.

7. **Baking Period:** Bake the apples for about 30 to 35 minutes, or until they are soft but not mushy, in a preheated oven.

8. **Serve:** After taking the baked apples out of the oven, let them cool a little. Warm them up and serve them on their own, or top with a drizzle of honey or a dollop of low-potassium vanilla yogurt, if preferred.

Estimated Preparation Time:

With baking time, Baked Apples with Cherries and Almonds should be completed in around 45 minutes.

Nutritional Value (about, per serving):

- 200 and 250 calories

- 2–3 grams of protein

- 5–6 grams of fiber

- 100–150 milligrams of potassium

- Cadmium: 50–60 mg

- Sodium: mg 0–10

- **Broccoli with lemon and garlic**

Ingredients:

- Four cups of newly cut broccoli florets

- Two minced garlic cloves

- One lemon's zest

- One lemon's juice

- Two tsp olive oil

- An alternative to salt (optional, to taste)

- To taste, freshly ground black pepper

Instructions:

1. **Cook the Broccoli:** Heat up a big saucepan of water until it boils. After adding them, blanch the broccoli florets for two to three minutes, or until they become brilliant green and start to soften.

2. **Cold Bath:** To halt the cooking process, quickly remove the blanched broccoli and submerge it in a bowl of icy water. This preserves the sharpness and vivid green color.

3. **Stir-fry the garlic:** Heat the olive oil in a big skillet over medium heat. When the garlic is fragrant but not browned, add the minced garlic and sauté it for about one minute.

4. **Stir in the broccoli:** After blanching the broccoli, drain and combine it with the garlic in a pan. Toss to coat the broccoli in the oil flavored with the garlic.

5. **Juice and Zest:** Squeeze the lemon juice evenly over the broccoli after removing the zest.

6. **Season to Taste**: If necessary, add freshly ground black pepper and a salt replacement to the dish's seasoning. Take a tiny bit at first and taste as needed.

7. **Cook and Serve:** Cook the broccoli in the skillet for a further two to three minutes, or until it's well cooked and flavored with garlic and lemon.

Estimated Preparation Time:

Broccoli with Garlic and Lemon takes around 15 to 20 minutes to prepare.

Nutritional Value (about, per serving):

- 80–100 calories

- 2–3 grams of protein

- 4–5 grams of fiber

- 200–250 milligrams of potassium

- Potassium: 40–50 mg

- Sodium 10–20 mg

Ingredients:

- One cup brown rice (choose a potassium-low type)

- Two cups of vegetable broth low in salt

- 1/2 cup finely chopped onions

- 1/2 cup finely sliced carrots

- 1/2 cup finely chopped celery

- Two minced garlic cloves

- Two tsp olive oil

- 1/4 cup chopped unsalted almonds (low phosphorus)

- 1/4 cup of raisins or dried cranberries

- Half a teaspoon of cumin powder

- An alternative to salt (optional, to taste)

- To taste, freshly ground black pepper

- Chopped fresh parsley, optional as a garnish

Instructions:

1. **After washing, toast the rice.**

- Use cold water to rinse the brown rice until the water turns clear. This gets rid of extra starch. Make sure to drain properly.

- Heat the olive oil in a big skillet over medium heat. After draining, add the rice and sauté it for three to four minutes, or until it starts to softly toast.

2. **Cook the Veggies:** Fill the skillet with the minced garlic, diced onion, carrots, and celery. Cook the veggies for a further three to four minutes, or until they start to get tender.

3. **Add the seasonings and broth:** Add the freshly ground black pepper, ground cumin, and salt replacement (if preferred) after adding the low-sodium vegetable broth.

4. **Simmer and Prepare:** Once the mixture reaches a boil, turn down the heat. For about 45 minutes, or until the rice is cooked through and has soaked up the liquid, simmer the mixture covered.

5. **Add the fruit and nuts:** Add the chopped unsalted almonds and dried cranberries or raisins five minutes before the rice is done. Simmer for the remaining amount of time.

6. **Serve and garnish:** Using a fork, fluff the brown rice pilaf and, if wanted, sprinkle with freshly chopped parsley.

Estimated Preparation Time:

The preparation of this Brown Rice Pilaf should take 60 to 70 minutes.

Nutritional Value (about, per serving):

- Between 200 and 250 calories

- 4–5 grams of protein

- 3–4 grams of fiber

- 150–200 milligrams of potassium

- 100–150 mg of phosphorus

- 100–150 mg of sodium

- Cranberry pecan rice pilaf

Ingredients:

- One cup of white rice (choose a potassium-low kind)

- Two cups of vegetable broth low in salt

- 1/2 cup finely chopped onions

- 1/2 cup finely chopped celery

- 1/2 cup finely sliced carrots

- Two minced garlic cloves

- Two tsp olive oil

- 1/4 cup chopped unsalted pecans (low phosphorus)

- 1/4 cup of low-potassium, unsweetened dried cranberries

- Half a teaspoon of cinnamon, ground

- An alternative to salt (optional, to taste)

- To taste, freshly ground black pepper

- Chopped fresh parsley, optional as a garnish

Instructions:

1. **Rinse the rice:** Use cold water to rinse the white rice until the water turns clear. This aids in removing too much starch. Make sure to drain properly.

2. **Heat up the rice:** Heat the olive oil in a big skillet over medium heat. When it's gently toasted, add the drained rice and sauté it for three to four minutes.

3. **Cook the Veggies:** Fill the skillet with the chopped onion, celery, carrots, and minced garlic. After 3–4 more minutes of sautéing, the veggies should start to soften.

4. **Add the seasonings and broth:** Add the freshly ground black pepper, ground cinnamon, and salt alternative (if preferred) after adding the low-sodium vegetable broth.

5. **Simmer and Prepare:** Once the mixture reaches a boil, turn down the heat. Once the rice is soft and has absorbed the liquid, cook it covered for 20 to 25 minutes.

6. **Add the fruit and nuts:** Add the chopped unsalted pecans and dried cranberries five minutes before the rice is done. Simmer for the remaining amount of time.

7. **Serve and garnish:** Using a fork, fluff the cranberry pecan rice pilaf. If preferred, sprinkle with freshly chopped parsley.

Estimated Preparation Time:

Making this Cranberry Pecan Rice Pilaf will take around 35 to 45 minutes.

Nutritional Value (about, per serving):

- 200 and 250 calories

- 3–4 grams of protein

- 2–3 grams of fiber

- 100–150 milligrams of potassium

- 60–70 mg of phosphorus

- 100–150 mg of sodium

- **Granola flavored with cinnamon, raisins, and apples**

Ingredients:

- Two cups of steel-cut oats

- 1/2 cup of low-phosphorus unsalted sunflower seeds

- 1/2 cup chopped unsalted almonds (low phosphorus)

- 1/2 cup chopped unsalted walnuts (low phosphorus)

- 1/2 cup chopped unsalted pecans (low phosphorus)

- 1/2 cup chopped dry apples (low potassium)

- Half a cup of raisins

- 1/4 cup honey or some other sugar

- One teaspoon of cinnamon powder

- 1/4 cup of applesauce without sugar

- Two tsp olive oil

- An alternative to salt (optional, to taste)

Instructions:

1. **Warm up the oven:** Set the oven temperature to 325°F, or 160°C.

2. **Blend the dry ingredients**: Combine the unsalted pecans, unsalted almonds, unsalted walnuts, unsalted sunflower seeds, and old-fashioned oats in a large mixing basin.

3. **Add the moist ingredients**: Combine the unsweetened applesauce, olive oil, ground cinnamon, honey or sugar replacement, and another bowl.

4. **Blend and Toss**: After pouring the wet mixture over the dry ingredients, toss to coat everything thoroughly. Add a small amount of salt substitute to taste, if desired.

5. **Line a baking sheet**: Evenly distribute the mixture onto a parchment paper-lined baking sheet.

6. **Cook**: Bake for 20 to 25 minutes, or until the granola is crunchy and golden brown, in a preheated oven. To guarantee uniform baking, stir it once or twice.

7. Once cooled, add fruit: After letting the granola cool, mix in the raisins and dried apples.

8. **Store**: After your kidney-friendly granola with raisins, apples, and cinnamon has fully cooled, put it in an airtight container.

Eat as a crunchy snack, as a topping for yogurt, or just by itself with milk.

Estimated Preparation Time:

It should take around 30 to 35 minutes to make this granola with raisins, apples, and cinnamon, including baking time.

Nutritional Value (about, per serving):

- 200 and 250 calories

- 5–6 grams of protein

- 3–4 grams of fiber

- 100–150 milligrams of potassium

- 100–150 mg of phosphorus

- Sodium: mg 0–10

- **Garlic and red pepper on green beans**

Ingredients:

- One pound of freshly cut green beans

- One red bell pepper, cut thinly

- Two minced garlic cloves

- Two tsp olive oil

- An alternative to salt (optional, to taste)

- To taste, freshly ground black pepper

- Chopped fresh parsley, optional as a garnish

Instructions:

1. **Green beans should be blanched**: Heat up a big saucepan of water until it boils. After adding the green beans, blanch them for three to four minutes, or until they become a brilliant green and start to soften.

2. **Cold Bath**: To halt the cooking process, immediately take the blanched green beans and place them in a dish of icy water. This keeps them fresh and vibrant green in color.

3. **Cook the Veggies**: Heat the olive oil in a big skillet over medium heat. When the red bell pepper begins to soften, add it and sauté it for two to three minutes.

4. **Add the green beans and garlic**:

- Add the minced garlic and cook for an additional minute after stirring.

- Fill the skillet with the blanched and drained green beans. Toss them with the garlic and sautéed red pepper to thoroughly warm them.

5. **Season to Taste**: If necessary, add freshly ground black pepper and a salt replacement to the dish's seasoning. Take a tiny bit at first and taste as needed.

6. **Serve and garnish**: Spoon the green beans, garlic, and red pepper onto a serving platter. Add freshly cut parsley as a garnish if you'd like.

Estimated Preparation Time:

Green beans with garlic and red pepper should be prepared in 20 to 25 minutes.

Nutritional Value (about, per serving):

- 80–100 calories

- 2–3 grams of protein

- 3–4 grams of fiber

- 200–250 milligrams of potassium

- Potassium: 20–30 mg

- Sodium: 0–10 mg

Ingredients:

- One cauliflower head, divided into florets

- Two tsp olive oil

- Grated Parmesan cheese, half a cup

- Two minced garlic cloves

- A teaspoon of thyme, dried

- An alternative to salt (optional, to taste)

- To taste, freshly ground black pepper

- Chopped fresh parsley, optional as a garnish

Instructions:

1. **Warm up the oven:** Set the oven's temperature to 425°F (220°C).

2. **Get the cauliflower ready**: Roughly chop the cauliflower into small pieces. Thoroughly rinse and drain them.

3. **Apply an olive oil coat**: Toss the cauliflower florets with olive oil in a big mixing basin until they're well coated.

4. **Include seasonings**: Garnish the cauliflower with the minced garlic and dry thyme. Add freshly ground black pepper and a sprinkle of salt replacement, if needed, to season. Toss to properly distribute the spices among the florets.

5. **In the oven, roast**: Arrange the seasoned cauliflower on a silicone baking mat or parchment paper-lined baking sheet.

6. **Cooking Timing**: Roast the cauliflower for 20 to 25 minutes in a preheated oven, stirring it once or twice to ensure equal cooking, or until it is soft and golden brown.

7. **Top with Parmesan cheese**: Remove the cauliflower from the oven five minutes or so before it's done, and then evenly sprinkle the grated Parmesan cheese on top.

8. **Complete Roasting**: Put the cauliflower back in the oven and continue to roast it until the cheese is melted and beginning to turn brown.

9. **Serve and garnish**: Take the Parmesan-roasted cauliflower out of the oven, and if you'd like, top with freshly chopped parsley. Serve as a delectable and kidney-friendly accompaniment.

Estimated Preparation Time:

After roasting, the recipe for Parmesan Roasted Cauliflower should take around 30 to 35 minutes to prepare.

Nutritional Value (Approximate, per serving):

- 100 and 150 calories

- 5–6 grams of protein

- 3–4 grams of fiber

- 300–350 milligrams of potassium

- 100–150 mg of phosphorus

Sodium: 200–250 mg

Ingredients:

- One pound of freshly cut green beans

- Two tsp olive oil

- Two minced garlic cloves

- An alternative to salt (optional, to taste)

- To taste, freshly ground black pepper

- Lemon zest, optional garnish

Instructions:

1. **Get the oven ready**: Set the oven's temperature to 425°F (220°C).

2. **Add olive oil and toss:** Toss the chopped green beans with olive oil in a big mixing bowl until they're well coated.

3. **Use garlic to season:** Evenly distribute the minced garlic by scattering it over the green beans and tossing them.

4. **Transfer to a baking sheet:** Spread out the spiced green beans in a single layer on a silicone baking mat or parchment paper-lined baking sheet.

5. **Add salt and pepper to taste:** Garnish the green beans with freshly ground black pepper and a pinch of salt substitute, if preferred.

6. **Bake in the Oven Roast:** Roast the green beans for 15 to 20 minutes, or until they are soft and beginning to brown. Toss them once or twice to ensure even cooking.

7. **Finish and Present:** You can add some fresh lemon zest to the Roasted Green Beans if you'd like.

Estimated Preparation Time:

After roasting, the recipe for Roasted Green Beans should take 20 to 25 minutes to prepare.

Nutritional Value (about, per serving):

- Between 60 and 80 calories

- 2–3 grams of protein

- 3–4 grams of fiber

- 200–250 milligrams of potassium

- Potassium: 20–30 mg

- Sodium: 0–10 mg

- Tasty buckwheat pilaf seasoned with roasted nuts

Ingredients:

- One cup of kasha, or buckwheat groats

- Two cups of vegetable broth low in salt

- 1/2 cup finely chopped onions

- 1/2 cup finely sliced carrots

- 1/2 cup finely chopped bell pepper, red or green

- Two minced garlic cloves

- Two tsp olive oil

- One teaspoon of cumin powder

- Half a teaspoon of coriander powder

- An alternative to salt (optional, to taste)

- To taste, freshly ground black pepper

- Chopped fresh parsley, optional as a garnish

Instructions:

1. **Wash the buckwheat**: After rinsing the buckwheat groats in cold water until the water runs clear, place them in a fine-mesh strainer. Make sure to drain properly.

2. **Buckwheat Toast**: In a dry skillet over medium heat, toast the rinsed buckwheat groats for 3–4 minutes, stirring frequently, until fragrant and just beginning to brown.

3. **Get the veggies ready**: Heat the olive oil in a different skillet over medium heat. Add the bell pepper, carrots, and onion, chopped. Sauté the vegetables for five to seven minutes, or until they start to get tender.

4. **Add the spices and garlic**: Add the ground coriander, cumin, and minced garlic and stir. Add another minute of sautéing.

5. **Blend and Cook**: Boil the low-sodium vegetable broth in a saucepan. When boiling, mix in the sautéed vegetables and toasted buckwheat groats. Add freshly ground black pepper and a sprinkle of salt replacement, if needed, to season.

6. **Cook and Simmer**: Lower the heat, place a lid on the saucepan, and simmer the buckwheat for ten to twelve minutes, or until it has become soft and absorbed the liquid.

7. **Fluff and Garnish**: Use a fork to fluff up the flavorful Buckwheat Pilaf. Add freshly cut parsley as a garnish if you'd like.

Estimated Preparation Time:

Savory Buckwheat Pilaf with Toasty Spices takes about 30 to 35 minutes to prepare.

Nutritional Value (about, per serving):

- 200 and 250 calories

- 6-7 grams of protein

- 4–5 grams of fiber

- 200–250 milligrams of potassium

- 150–200 mg of phosphorus

- 100–150 mg of sodium

- Wild rice pilaf topped with apples and cranberries

Ingredients:

– One cup of wild rice

- Two cups of vegetable broth low in salt

- 1/2 cup finely chopped onions

- 1/2 cup finely chopped apples (select an apple variety low in potassium)

- 1/4 cup of low-potassium, unsweetened dried cranberries

- Two minced garlic cloves

- Two tsp olive oil

- 1/4 cup chopped unsalted almonds (low phosphorus)

- Half a teaspoon of cinnamon, ground

- An alternative to salt (optional, to taste)

- To taste, freshly ground black pepper

- Chopped fresh parsley, optional as a garnish

Instructions:

1. Clean and Cook Wild Rice:

- Use cold water to rinse the wild rice until the water turns clear. Make sure to drain properly.

- Place the low-sodium vegetable broth and rinsed wild rice in a saucepan. After bringing it to a boil, lower the heat, cover it, and simmer the rice for 45 to 60 minutes, or until it is soft and the liquid has been absorbed. Remove any extra liquid.

2. **Get the apples and vegetables ready:**

- Heat the olive oil in a skillet over medium heat while the rice is simmering. When the onion is translucent, add it and sauté it for five to seven minutes.

- Add the ground cinnamon, chopped apples, dried cranberries, and minced garlic. The apples should soften slightly after another two to three minutes of sautéing.

3. **Blend and Flavor:**

- Put the cooked wild rice and the sautéed apple, cranberry, and onion mixture into a big mixing bowl. Toss to evenly combine.

- Add a dash of freshly ground black pepper and salt substitute, if preferred. To suit your taste.

4. **Finish and Serve:** You can add some freshly chopped parsley to your kidney-friendly wild rice pilaf along with some cranberries and apples.

Estimated Preparation Time:

Including the time for the rice to cook, preparing Wild Rice Pilaf with Cranberries and Apples should take approximately 75-90 minutes.

Nutritional Value (about, per serving):

- 200 and 250 calories

- 5–6 grams of protein

- 4–5 grams of fiber

- 150–200 milligrams of potassium

- 100–150 mg of phosphorus

- 100–150 mg of sodium

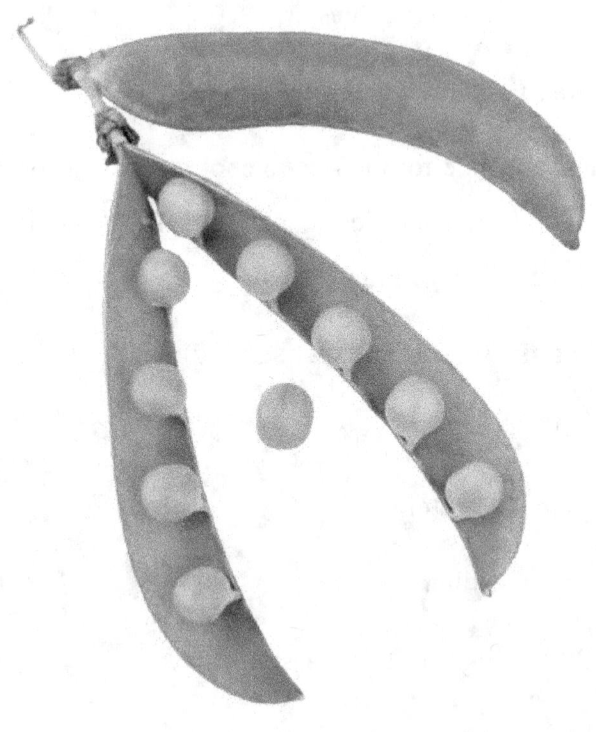

CHAPTER SIX

Snacks and Starters: Enhance the Experience

-Bag of bread sticks

Ingredients:

- One package of premade, low-sodium, low-phosphorus breadsticks that are good for the kidneys

- Spray with olive oil (to brush)

- Garlic powder (for flavor; optional)

- Dried parsley (for flavoring; optional)

Instructions:

1. **Warm up the oven**: Set the oven temperature to 375–400°F (190-200°C), as recommended by the breadstick box.

2. **Get the breadsticks ready**: Open the packet of premade kidney-friendly breadsticks and place them on a baking pan.

3. **Apply an olive oil brush**: Lightly drizzle little olive oil over each breadstick. This will aid in their browning and crisping during baking.

4. **Season (Selective):** For added taste, you can, if you'd like, sprinkle some dried parsley and garlic powder on top of the breadsticks.

5. **Cook**: After preheating the oven, place the baking sheet with the breadsticks inside and bake them for the recommended amount of time (usually 10 to 15 minutes), or until they are crispy and golden brown.

Let the breadsticks cool on a plate or a wire rack for a few minutes. You may serve your kidney-friendly Bag of Bread Sticks with your preferred kidney-friendly dip or as a delicious snack.

Estimated Preparation Time:

Using pre-made breadsticks makes creating a Bag of Bread Sticks fast—about 15 to 20 minutes.

Nutritional Value (per serving):

The exact brand and kind of breadsticks you use will affect the nutritional content. For comprehensive nutritional information, consult the packaging.

- rice cakes topped with chopped peppers or cucumbers and low-fat cream cheese

Ingredients:

- Rice cakes; select low-phosphorus, low-sodium types.

- Low-fat cheese with cream

- Slicing a cucumber thinly

- Thinly sliced bell peppers (choose a kind with low potassium content).

- Chopped fresh chives (optional garnish)

- An alternative to salt (optional, to taste)

- To taste, freshly ground black pepper

Instructions:

1. Get the rice cakes ready by: Arrange the rice cakes on a spotlessly tidy surface.

2. Distribute Cream Cheese: Top each rice cake with a layer of reduced-fat cream cheese.

3. Include peppers or cucumbers: Arrange thin slices of bell peppers or cucumber on top of the cream cheese. Using any or both will rely on your own choice.

4. Season (Optional): Add freshly ground black pepper and a sprinkle of salt replacement, if preferred.

5. Accessory (Optional): Top with finely chopped fresh chives for taste and a pop of color.

Arrange on a dish or platter your kidney-friendly Rice Cakes with Low-Fat Cream Cheese and Sliced Peppers or Cucumber. Serve as a healthy, kidney-friendly appetizer or snack.

Estimated Preparation Time:

It just takes ten to fifteen minutes to make Rice Cakes with Low-Fat Cream Cheese and Sliced Peppers or Cucumbers.

Nutritional Value (about, per serving):

The particular brands and amounts you use will affect the nutritional values. Although the potassium and phosphorus content of this snack is normally modest, it's crucial to select cream cheese and rice cakes that are low in both salt and phosphorus.

- **Low-fat hummus and carrot sticks**

Ingredients:

- Low-fat hummus (homemade or from the supermarket)

- A variety of kidney-friendly veggies, such celery sticks, bell pepper strips, cucumber slices, and carrot sticks, for dipping

- Chopped fresh parsley (optional for garnish)

- Lemon wedges, if desired, as a garnish

- An alternative to salt (optional, to taste)

- To taste, freshly ground black pepper

Instructions:

1. **Get the hummus ready**: If you're using reduced-fat hummus from the grocery, move it to a serving dish. If you're preparing your own hummus, put it in a bowl and use your favorite recipe.

2. **Get the veggies ready**: Prepare kidney-friendly veggies for dipping, such as bell pepper strips, cucumber slices, carrot sticks, and celery sticks. Wash and chop them. Place them next to the hummus or on a serving plate.

3. **Season (Selective):** You may optionally add freshly ground black pepper and a sprinkle of salt replacement to the hummus to season it. For extra taste, squeeze some fresh lemon juice from the lemon wedges and drizzle it over.

4. **Accessory (Optional):** To add some color and flavor to the hummus, sprinkle chopped fresh parsley on top.

Arrange the veggie stick plate and the dish of hummus on your serving table. Serve as a filling and kidney-friendly snack. Dip the veggie sticks into the hummus to have a tasty and healthy snack.

Estimated Preparation Time:

It just takes ten to fifteen minutes to make Reduced-Fat Hummus with Vegetable Sticks, depending on whether you use homemade or store-bought hummus.

Nutritional Value (about, per serving):

The particular brands and amounts you use will affect the nutritional values. Kidney-friendly snacks like this one are typically okay, but be sure to select low-fat hummus and low-potassium veggies for pairing.

- Renal Diet Style: Appetizer Artistry

- Avocado deviled eggs

Ingredients:

- Six big eggs

- One mature avocado

- One or two teaspoons reduced-fat mayo

- One teaspoon of mustard dijon

- A tsp of freshly squeezed lemon juice

- An alternative to salt (optional, to taste)

- To taste, freshly ground black pepper

- Paprika (optional garnish)

- Chopped fresh chives (optional garnish)

Instructions:

1. **Boil the Eggs Hard**: Put the eggs in a pan with water on top of them. After bringing the water to a boil, lower the heat to a gentle simmer and let it cook for ten to twelve minutes.

Take the eggs off of the heat source and place them right away in an ice bath to cool.

2. **Split and peel the eggs**: Peel and cut the eggs in half lengthwise after they have cooled. After removing the yolks, transfer them to a mixing dish.

3. **Get the avocado ready**: Halve the ripe avocado, remove the pit, and extract the flesh with a spoon. In the mixing dish with the egg yolks, add the avocado.

4. **Blend**: Mash the avocado and egg yolks together with a fork until a homogeneous mixture forms. To get the right consistency, you can add one or two teaspoons of low-fat mayonnaise if necessary.

5. **Add Taste**: Add the Dijon mustard and lemon juice, and season with a dash of salt replacement and freshly ground black pepper, if preferred. Taste and adjust the seasoning.

6. **Pour Egg Whites into Them**:

- Spoon or pipette the avocado and yolk mixture into the hollowed-out egg whites.

- For a vibrant garnish, feel free to top with chopped fresh chives or a small pinch of paprika.

- Transfer your Avocado Deviled Eggs to a platter for presentation.

- Serve as a delicious and kidney-friendly snack or appetizer.

Estimated Preparation Time:

It should take between 30 to 35 minutes to make avocado deviled eggs, including cooking the eggs and assembling them.

Nutritional Value (per serving):

The exact brands and amounts you use will determine the differences in nutritional content. Generally speaking, this dish is kidney-friendly; nevertheless, utilize low-potassium and low-phosphorus components.

- Baba Ghanaoush

Ingredients:

- Two eggplants, medium

- Two minced garlic cloves

- Two tablespoons of sesame paste, or tahini.

- Two tsp freshly squeezed lemon juice

- Two tsp olive oil

- A taste-tested salt replacement

- To taste, freshly ground black pepper

- Chopped fresh parsley, optional as a garnish

- Paprika, as an optional garnish

Instructions:

1. **Make the eggplants roast**: Set the oven temperature to 400°F, or 200°C. After putting the eggplants on a baking sheet, roast them for 40 to 45 minutes, rotating them halfway through, or until the flesh is tender and the skin is browned. If you want a smokey taste, you may also roast the eggplants over an open flame.

2. **Peel and Cool**: Take the roasted eggplants out of the grill or oven and allow them to cool. After it has cooled, remove the burnt outer layer to reveal the tender inner layer.

3. **Fry the eggplant**: To make a smooth puree, put the peeled eggplant flesh in a basin and mash it with a fork or potato masher. Throw away any big seeds.

4. **Add the components**:

- Mix the mashed eggplant with olive oil, tahini, fresh lemon juice, and chopped garlic. Toss them together thoroughly.

- Add freshly ground black pepper and a salt replacement to your Baba Ghanoush. Taste and adjust the seasoning.

- To let the flavors to merge, cover the dish and chill the Baba Ghanoush for at least one or two hours.

- Garnish with freshly chopped parsley and paprika, if like, before serving.

- Pair your homemade Baba Ghanoush with pita bread, crackers, or raw vegetable sticks as a kidney-friendly dip.

Estimated Preparation Time:

When making Baba Ghanoush, allow 60 to 70 minutes for chilling and roasting.

Nutritional Value (about, per serving):

The exact brands and amounts you use will determine the differences in nutritional content. In general, baba ghanoush is kidney-friendly; however, make sure the tahini and other components are minimal in phosphorus and salt.

- **Stuffed mushrooms with basil pesto**

Ingredients:

- Twelve huge white mushrooms with their stems removed and cleaned

- 1/3 cup homemade or store-bought basil pesto

– 1/3 cup of cream cheese without fat

- Two tablespoons of low-phosphorus grated Parmesan cheese

- One minced garlic clove

- A tsp of olive oil

- An alternative to salt (optional, to taste)

- To taste, freshly ground black pepper

- Fresh basil leaves, optional as a garnish

Instructions:

1. **Warm up the oven**: Set the oven temperature to 375°F, or 190°C.

2. **Get the mushrooms ready**: To make a hollow hole for the filling, carefully remove the mushroom stems. Chop the mushroom stems finely and reserve.

3. **Get the Filling Ready**: Combine the chopped mushroom stems, low-fat cream cheese, grated Parmesan cheese, minced garlic, and basil pesto in a mixing dish. Blend until the filling is smooth and creamy.

4. **The Mushroom Stuff**: Stuff the pesto and cream cheese mixture into each mushroom cap using a spoon or tiny spatula. Gently press the filler down.

5. **Olive oil drizzled on top**: Arrange the filled mushrooms onto a sheet pan. Pour a small amount of olive oil onto the top of every filled mushroom.

6. **Season**:

- Add freshly ground black pepper and a sprinkle of salt replacement, if preferred, to the filled mushrooms.

- Bake the stuffed mushrooms for 20 to 25 minutes in a preheated oven, or until the filling is golden brown and the mushrooms are soft.

- Garnish with fresh basil leaves for presentation and taste, if preferred.

- Arrange your stuffed mushrooms with basil pesto on a serving plate.

- Serve as a tasty and kidney-friendly side dish or appetizer.

Estimated Preparation Time:

With baking time, the preparation of Basil Pesto Stuffed Mushrooms should take around 30 to 35 minutes.

Nutritional Value (about, per serving):

The exact brands and amounts you use will determine the differences in nutritional content. Overall, this dish is kidney-friendly; however, be sure the components are minimal in phosphorus and salt.

- **Grilled pineapple**

Ingredients:

- One fresh pineapple, cut into rounds or wedges after being peeled and cored.

- One tablespoon honey (or your preferred kidney-friendly sweetener, if preferred)

- One teaspoon of ground cinnamon, if desired

- Olive oil spray (optional for grilling)

- Fresh mint leaves (optional garnish)

Instructions:

1. **Get the pineapple ready**: Peel the pineapple and cut off the core first. Depending on your preference, cut the pineapple into rounds or wedges.

2. **Add-on Sweetener**: Drizzle honey or your favorite kidney-friendly sweetener over the pineapple slices if you'd like to add a little sweetness. For extra taste, you may also add ground cinnamon. You can skip this step, especially if you like the pineapple's natural sweetness.

3. **Warm up the grill:** Set the temperature of your grill to medium-high. If you like, you may use a little olive oil spray to keep the grill grates from sticking.

4. **The pineapple is grilled**: Straightforwardly place the pineapple slices on the barbecue grates. Grill the pineapple

for two to three minutes on each side, or until grill marks appear and it begins to caramelize.

5. **Accessory (Optional):** To add a pop of freshness, you may optionally garnish your grilled pineapple with mint leaves.

- Spread out the grilled pineapple on a plate for serving.

- Take advantage of the sweet and smokey aromas of your Grilled Pineapple and enjoy it as a dessert or side dish that is kidney-friendly.

Estimated Preparation Time:

Grilled pineapple should be prepared in 15 to 20 minutes.

Nutritional Value (about, per serving):

The exact brands and amounts you use will determine the differences in nutritional content. In general, grilled pineapple is safe for your kidneys, especially if it's not too sweetened.

Ingredients:

- One 15-ounce can (drained and rinsed) of chickpeas (garbanzo beans)

- Two minced garlic cloves

- 1/4 cup sesame paste, or tahini

- 1/4 cup freshly squeezed lemon juice (about one big lemon)

- Two tsp olive oil

- Half a teaspoon of cumin powder

- A taste-tested salt replacement

- To taste, freshly ground black pepper

- Water (as required for uniformity).

- Paprika (optional garnish)

- Chopped fresh parsley (optional garnish)

Instructions:

1. **Get the chickpeas ready**: Empty and thoroughly wash the chickpeas with cold water.

2. **Mix Elements Together**: Place the chickpeas, finely chopped garlic, tahini, lemon juice, olive oil, cumin powder, sprinkle of salt alternative, and freshly ground black pepper in a food processor.

3. **Combine**: Blend the ingredients thoroughly using a food processor. To make sure all of the ingredients are well combined, you might need to pause and scrape down the food processor's edges.

4. **Modify Uniformity**: You may gradually add water, one tablespoon at a time, to the hummus if it's too thick, until you have the right consistency.

5. **Tasty Seasoning**: Taste the hummus and adjust the flavor if necessary with more lemon juice, freshly ground black pepper, or salt replacement.

6. **Optional Garnish**: For extra taste and appearance, you may optionally top your hummus with chopped fresh parsley and a sprinkling of paprika.

- Transfer the hummus to a dish for serving.

- Serve your homemade hummus as a delicious spread or dip, or with pita bread and fresh veggies.

Estimated Preparation Time:

Classic hummus takes ten to fifteen minutes to prepare.

Nutritional Value (about, per serving):

The exact brands and amounts you use will determine the differences in nutritional content. Overall, this meal is suitable for those with kidneys; however, ensure that the tahini and other components are low in phosphorus and salt.

- Hummus with peanut butter

Ingredients:

- One 15-ounce can (drained and rinsed) of chickpeas (garbanzo beans)

- Two tablespoons of unsweetened peanut butter

- Two minced garlic cloves

- 1/4 cup freshly squeezed lemon juice (about one big lemon)

- Two tsp olive oil

- Half a teaspoon of cumin powder

- A taste-tested salt replacement

- To taste, freshly ground black pepper

- Water (as required for uniformity).

- Chopped peanuts (optional garnish)

- Fresh cilantro leaves (optional garnish)

Instructions:

1. **Get the chickpeas ready**: Empty and thoroughly wash the chickpeas with cold water.

2. **Mix Elements Together**: Place the chickpeas, peanut butter, minced garlic, fresh lemon juice, olive oil, ground cumin, freshly ground black pepper, and a little amount of salt replacement in a food processor.

3. **Combine**: Blend the ingredients thoroughly using a food processor. To make sure all of the ingredients are well combined, you might need to pause and scrape down the food processor's edges. You may gradually add water, one tablespoon at a time, to the hummus if it's too thick, until you have the right consistency.

4. **Tasty Seasoning**: Taste the hummus and adjust the flavor if necessary with more lemon juice, freshly ground black pepper, or salt replacement.

5. **Optional Garnish**:

- If you'd like, add more flavor and visual appeal to your Peanut Butter Hummus by adding chopped peanuts and fresh cilantro leaves.

- Transfer the hummus to a dish for serving.

- Serve your homemade peanut butter hummus as a unique and tasty spread or dip, or with pita bread and fresh veggies.

Estimated Preparation Time:

It should take ten to fifteen minutes to make peanut butter hummus.

Nutritional Value (about, per serving):

The exact brands and amounts you use will determine the differences in nutritional content. Though make sure your peanut butter and other components are minimal in salt and phosphorus, this dish is typically kidney-friendly.

Ingredients:

- One pound of freshly cut spears of asparagus that fit the container.

- Two cups vinegar (white)

- Two cups of water

- Two peeled and slightly crushed garlic cloves

- Two tablespoons of salt alternative

- One teaspoon sugar or your preferred kidney-friendly sweetener

- One-half teaspoon ground black pepper

- 1/2 teaspoon of optionally spicy red pepper flakes

- 2–3 fresh dill sprigs (optional)

- Lidded, sterilised glass jars

Instructions:

1. **Get the asparagus ready**: Carefully wash the asparagus, then clip any tough ends so they will fit into the glass jars

that you have sterilized. To make them fit, trim them to the appropriate length.

2. **Get the brine ready**: Combine white vinegar, water, garlic, sugar (or a kidney-friendly sweetener), salt alternative, black peppercorns, and red pepper flakes (if desired) in a pot. After bringing the mixture to a boil, simmer it for a short while.

3. **Jar Sterilization**: Make sure your glass jars and lids are thoroughly sanitized while the brine is cooking. To do this, you may either put them through a dishwasher or submerge them in hot water for a short while.

4. **Assemble Jars**: Pack the sterilized jars with the asparagus spears and fresh dill sprigs, if using.

5. **Transfer the Warm Brine**: Gently fill the jars with the hot brine mixture, making sure the asparagus is well submerged. Give the tops of the jars a headspace of approximately 1/2 inch.

6. **Close the Jars**: Tightly fit the sterilized lids onto the jars.

7. **Classy**: Let the jars cool until they reach room temperature.

8. **Keep cold**: After cooling, keep the pickled asparagus in the fridge for two to three days to let the flavors meld. Store the pickled asparagus in the refrigerator for many weeks.

9. **Serve**: Serve your homemade pickled asparagus as an appetizer, garnish, or tangy, crisp side dish.

Estimated Preparation Time:

Refrigeration time is not included in the estimated 30–40 minutes needed to make pickled asparagus.

Nutritional Value (about, per serving):

The exact brands and amounts you use will determine the differences in nutritional content. Though make sure your components are minimal in salt, this dish is typically kidney-friendly.

CHAPTER SEVEN

Quench Your Thirst: Kidney-Safe Drinks - Hydration Tricks

Without a doubt, maintaining adequate hydration is essential to a renal diet. For those who have worries about the health of their kidneys, consider these water tips:

1. **Monitor Fluid Intake**: Keep a careful eye on the amount of fluids you consume each day. Based on your unique kidney condition, your dietician or healthcare professional can offer you customized recommendations. Keep in mind that drinking too much liquids might cause fluid retention and put more strain on the kidneys.

2. **Strike a Balance between Fluid Restrictions and Thirst**: It's critical to find a way to both quench your thirst and control your intake of fluids. To find out how much fluid you should be consuming, see your doctor or a dietician.

3. **Regulate Your Sodium Intake**: Consuming too much sodium might make you more thirsty and retain more moisture. Avoid processed and high-sodium meals to reduce

your sodium consumption. Choose low-sodium or fresh alternatives.

4. **Select the Correct Beverages**: When it comes to staying hydrated, not all drinks are created equal. Although water is usually the best option, other options include ice pops, herbal teas, and clear broths that can also help you stay hydrated and relieve your thirst. Avoid or use sugary and caffeinated drinks sparingly.

5. **Measure and Monitor**: To keep track of your fluid consumption, use a measuring cup or bottle. This makes sure you don't go over your suggested daily allowance.

6. **Include Hydrating Foods in Meals**: To help you reach your fluid requirements, include hydrating foods in your meals, such as watermelon, cucumbers, and lettuce, which are high in water content.

7. **Handle Medication**: Recognize how your drugs affect your fluid balance if you are taking any for your kidney disease. Observe the advice of your healthcare professional with regard to taking your medications and staying hydrated.

8. **Speak with a Dietitian:** A qualified nutritionist with expertise in renal nutrition may design a personalized meal

plan and hydration strategy that takes into consideration your individual requirements. They may offer insightful advice on keeping renal health and fluid balance.

9. **Remain Cool in Hot Weather**: Be especially mindful of your fluid balance in hot weather. To reduce fluid loss via sweating, stay in a cool atmosphere, wear light clothing, and refrain from strenuous physical activity.

10. **Regular Monitoring**: As directed by your healthcare professional, keep a regular eye on your blood pressure and kidney function. Your fluid management can be guided by adjustments to these factors. Your kidney health can be greatly impacted by how well you hydrate.

- Drinking Our Way to Well-Being: Renal Diet Drinks

The selection of drinks is important in a renal diet to maintain kidney function and handle some dietary limitations. Some safe and typically kidney-friendly drinks for those with renal disease include:

1. **Water**: Water is the best option for staying hydrated without putting too much strain on the kidneys. It is necessary to keep the kidneys functioning properly.

2. **Herbal Teas**: The majority of herbal teas, including hibiscus, mint, and chamomile, are low in potassium and naturally caffeine-free. They can be a tasty and refreshing option.

3. **Fruit-Flavored Water**: For a cool twist, add slices of kidney-friendly fruits to your water, such as cucumber, lemon, lime, or berries.

4. **Decaffeinated Coffee**: Choose decaf varieties if you're a coffee enthusiast. Potassium and phosphorus content of decaf coffee is often lower than that of normal coffee.

5. **Decaffeinated Tea**: Decaffeinated teas might be good options. Examples include herbal teas and decaf black tea. Compared to their caffeinated equivalents, they frequently have lower potassium and phosphorus contents.

6. **Lemonade or Limeade**: A tangy, refreshing, and kidney-friendly beverage is homemade lemonade or limeade with no sugar.

7. **Apple Juice**: Compared to other fruit juices like orange or tomato juice, clear apple juice has less potassium.

8. **Cranberry Juice**: Because of its acidic flavor and decreased potassium level, unsweetened cranberry juice might be an excellent option when consumed in moderation.

9. **Ginger Ale**: Compared to cola and other beverages, ginger ale frequently has less potassium and phosphorus. As an alternative, look for sparkling water with a ginger taste or minimal sodium content.

10. **Rice Milk**: Unsweetened rice milk is a low-phosphorus choice for people who require a dairy substitute. Make sure to select kinds free of additives derived from phosphorus.

11. **Almond milk** (in moderation): An alternative milk with less phosphorus is unsweetened almond milk. It is crucial to use it sparingly, though.

12. **Homemade Smoothies**: Use ice, unsweetened yogurt or milk substitutes, low-potassium fruits, and kidney-friendly ingredients to make kidney-friendly smoothies. Avert fruits heavy in potassium, such as bananas.

13. **Carbonated Water**: An easy-to-drink, hydrated option is plain, unflavored carbonated water. Usually, it has no sodium, potassium, or phosphorus.

14. **Clear Broths**: If your appetite is down, low-sodium or homemade bone broth might be a warm and comforting choice.

15. **Homemade Fruit Sorbet**: Using low-potassium fruits and a sweetener that is healthy for kidneys, make your own fruit sorbet.

CHAPTER EIGHT

Eating Beyond Your Kitchen: Dining Out and Celebrations

- Using Your Confidence to Navigate Restaurants,

It takes some preparation and knowledge to eat out while on a renal diet, but it is very feasible.

1. **Conduct Pre-Project Research:** If at all feasible, browse a restaurant's menu online before selecting one. Seek alternatives that fit your dietary requirements.

2. **Make an Informed Restaurant Selection**: Choose eateries with a wide selection of meals; this will increase your possibilities for finding kidney-friendly fare. Certain cuisines, such as Japanese or Mediterranean, typically provide more appropriate options.

3. **Express Your Nutritional Requirements**: Never be afraid to let your server know about any dietary requirements. Inquire about the ingredients and cooking

methods used in the dishes. Special dietary preferences can be accommodated by many establishments.

4. **Request Adjustments**: Ask that recipes be changed to make them kidney-friendly. Request sauces and dressings on the side, for instance, or ask for your food to be cooked with less salt.

5. **Regulate Phosphorus and Sodium**: Pay attention to foods heavy in phosphorus and salt. Steer clear of foods that contain processed meats, cheese, or some sauces since they may be high in phosphorus and salt.

6. **Opt for Easy Preparations**: Simpler foods, such as those that are grilled or broiled, are frequently better selections. Avert fried or breaded meals as they may include elevated levels of phosphorus and salt.

7. **Choose Lean Proteins Instead**: Choose lean protein sources like tofu, turkey, fish, or chicken. They usually include less potassium and phosphorus.

8. **Observe the Portion Sizes**: Be mindful of serving sizes. The portions in restaurants may be rather substantial, so think about splitting the meal with someone else or packing leftovers to go.

9. **Forego or alter the appetizers**: Appetizers with high salt and phosphorus content include nachos and onion rings. Instead, go for a straightforward salad or a low-sodium soup.

10. **Watch Out for Stealth Sodium**: Be wary of foods that have sauces, dressings, or condiments on them since they may conceal high salt content. Ask to have them on the side or for low-sodium substitutes.

11. **Regulate Your Fluid Consumption**: Pay attention to what you drink if you're following a diet low in fluids. In moderation, stick to water, herbal tea, or a clear soda.

12. **Dessert Substitutes**: If available, select fruit or sorbet for dessert. Steer clear of high-potassium foods like bananas, almonds, and chocolate.

13. **Find Out About Kidney-Friendly Substitutes**: Some eateries could provide kidney-friendly selections or be open to changing their cuisine to meet your dietary requirements.

14. **Always Carry a List of Food Limitations**: To make sure your needs are met, think about bringing a little card or letter with your dietary limitations that you can show the waiter.

15. **Apply Restraint**: Enjoying a pleasure now and again is OK, but moderation is essential. Consider the total amount of nutrients you consume.

- **Joyous Gathering with Renal Flair**

Following a renal diet does not exclude enjoying festive events, in fact, it may even be fun.

1. **Make a Plan**: Planning is essential. Talk to your healthcare practitioner and nutritionist about your food choices and limits before the celebrations begin. They may offer insightful advice and recommendations that are appropriate for the situation.

2. **Interaction Is Crucial**: Let the host or hostess know in advance about any food restrictions you may have while attending get-togethers or family celebrations. This can assist them in making kidney-friendly dishes.

3. **Propose to Help Out**: Make a kidney-friendly meal that you can eat and share with others if you're bringing food to a potluck or other event.

4. **Select Astute Initiators**: Select appetizers in accordance with your dietary requirements. A kidney-friendly dip, unsalted almonds, or platters of fresh fruit or vegetables can all be excellent options.

5. **Conscientious Main Dishes**: Choose lean protein alternatives for the main dish, such as fish, poultry, or turkey. Steer clear of processed meats as they are often heavy in salt.

6. **Handle the Season**: Ask to have your meal cooked with less salt, or use spices and herbs low in sodium to flavor your cuisine.

7. **Restrict Foods High in Potassium**: Pay attention to foods high in potassium, such as potatoes, tomatoes, and bananas. Choose other options or eat these meals sparingly.

8. **Control of Portion**: Festive feasts frequently have a lot of food. Limit serving quantities to prevent overindulging.

9. **Staying Hydrated Is Vital**: Continue adhering to any appropriate fluid limits. Select low-sodium or low-potassium drinks, and keep a careful eye on how much fluid you're consuming.

10. **Sides Suitable for Kidneys**: Make kidney-friendly side dishes, including rice pilaf made with low-potassium components, a fresh salad, or roasted vegetables.

11. **Modest Sweet Treats**: Delight in dessert sparingly. Desserts made with a kidney-safe sweetener, sorbet, or a tiny piece of low-potassium fruit pie can all be alternatives.

12. **Keep Moving**: Include some physical activities in your celebrations, such a stroll after dinner or enjoyable outdoor games with loved ones.

13. **Mentality Counts**: Pay more attention to the happiness of spending time with family and friends than just the cuisine. The purpose of festive events is to celebrate and make memories with one another.

14. **Prepare a Menu for Any Leftovers**: In the days after the celebration, think about how to use any leftovers to make kidney-friendly meals.

15. **Speak with Your Nutritionist**: Your nutritionist may assist you in developing a menu that complies with your dietary requirements and includes ideas for special occasions.

16. **Calm Is the Key**: Recall that indulging in a treat on noteworthy events is totally acceptable. Just watch your total nutritional intake and portion sizes.

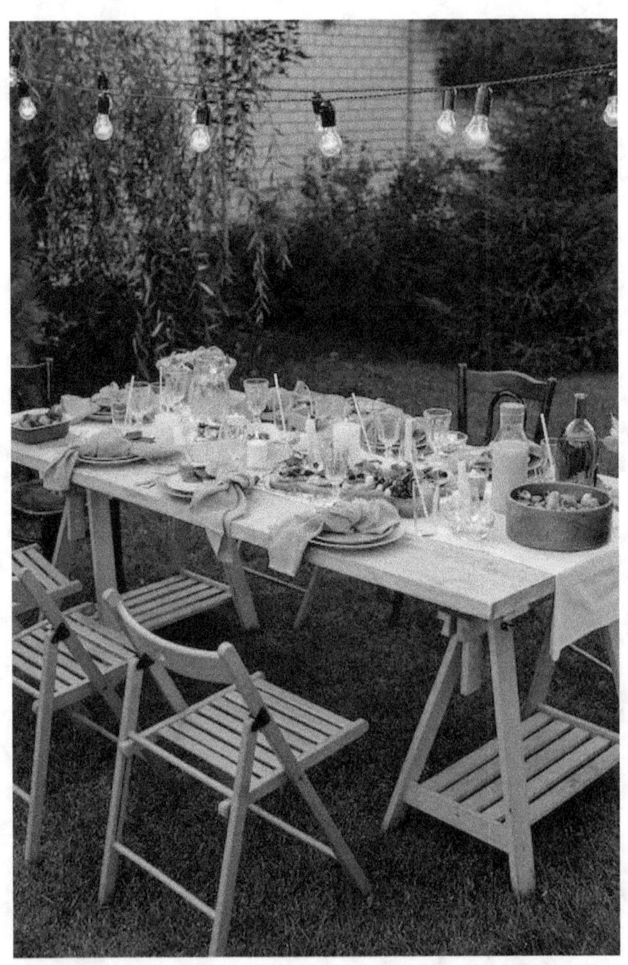

CHAPTER NINE

Setting the Course: Moderation and Meal Planning

- Weekly Dinner Masterpieces

For people on a renal diet, meal planning is a useful tactic. It enables you to arrange and plan your meals while adhering to your dietary requirements. This is a weekly meal plan for preparing meals on a renal diet:

Week 1: Organizing and Purchasing

1. **Evaluate Dietary Restrictions**: To learn more about your individual dietary requirements, speak with a dietician or your healthcare physician. Establish your daily limitations for salt, potassium, phosphorus, and protein.

2. **Make a Meal Plan**: Plan out your meals for the coming week, including breakfast, lunch, supper, and snacks. Make kidney-friendly products and meals your main focus.

3. **Create a Shopping List**: Using your meal plan as a guide, make a thorough list of items to buy that are both kidney-friendly and portion-appropriate.

4. **Shop Wisely**: Pay close attention to the labels of foods you purchase to determine the amount of phosphorus, potassium, and sodium. Select low-potassium, low-phosphorus, and low-sodium choices.

Week 2: Freezing and Batch Cooking

5. **Batch Cooking**: Make bigger batches of kidney-friendly meals like veggies, grains, and lean meats over the weekends. Cook the beans, rice, and simple chicken so they may be used in a variety of recipes.

6. **Portion and Freeze**: Divide prepared meals into serving-sized portions and store them in the freezer. This lessens the need to prepare every day by enabling you to have ingredients available for future meals.

Week 3: Examining Recipes

7. **Try New meals**: To spice up your eating plan, try out some new kidney-friendly meals. Every day, try a different meal to see what you like.

8. **Adjust and Modify**: Try modifying a recipe to suit your needs if the amount of sodium, potassium, or phosphorus isn't quite correct.

Week 4: Putting the Plan into Action

9. **Cook with Confidence**: Start by utilizing the supplies and prepared components from the freezer and according to your meal plan. Daily food preparation will become more efficient as a result.

10. **Portion Control**: Be mindful of serving sizes to make sure you don't eat more than you need to each day.

11. **Track and Modify**: Maintain a food journal to keep tabs on your daily consumption and evaluate how well your meal plan fits into your nutritional objectives. Make any required modifications.

Ongoing: Constantly Preparing Meals

12. **Repeat and Improve**: Stick to the meal planning schedule you set up during the first month. This will assist in maintaining diet consistency.

13. **Consult Your nutritionist**: Have regular meetings with your nutritionist to discuss your nutritional progress and to discuss any adjustments that need be made to your menu.

14. **Remain Hydrated**: Do not forget to follow your doctor's recommendations on how much liquids you consume. Keep an eye on how much liquids you drink each day and adhere to the suggested guidelines.

15. **Be Aware of Medication**: Talk to your doctor to make sure there are no contraindications to any drugs before making dietary decisions because certain medications may interact with certain foods.

- Portion Control

Managing dietary limits and preserving kidney health need you to become an expert in portion management on your renal diet. Here are some tips to assist you in successfully regulating portion sizes:

1. **Use Measuring Tools**: Purchase a kitchen scale and measuring cups. With the use of these gadgets, you can precisely gauge the serving sizes of different meals and make sure your intake stays within your allotted limits.

2. **Recognize Common Portion Sizes**: Acquaint yourself with typical serving sizes for everyday items. A deck of cards, for instance, is about the size of three ounces of beef or chicken.

3. **Carefully Plate Your Food**: Use smaller bowls and plates to help you automatically regulate portion amounts. This reduces the amount of food on the plate while giving the impression that it is full.

4. **Divide Your Dish**: Assign parts to your plate mentally. Distribute the platter such that non-starchy veggies make up half, lean protein makes up quarter, and kidney-friendly starch makes up the remaining quarter.

5. **Snacks Prior to Portion**: As soon as you bring them home, divide them into single-serving quantities if you're a snacker. This facilitates grabbing a food that has been portioned out.

6. **Steer clear of buffet dining**: Take care not to fill your plate to the brim during family-style meals or buffets. Before determining whether you want more, start with smaller servings and wait.

7. **Distribute Restaurant Plates**: If you're dining with someone, think about splitting an entrée. Restaurant servings frequently exceed what is required for a single meal.

8. **Make a Takeout Container Request**: If a restaurant serves a large quantity, ask for a takeout container right away and freeze half of the food for later use.

9. **Carefully Read Labels**: Read food labels carefully to determine serving sizes and nutritional information. Adapt your portions according to the given information.

10. **Make Mindful Food Choices**: Take your time and enjoy your meal. Give the tastes and textures some time to settle in. By doing this, overeating may be avoided.

11. **Sip Water Prior to Eating**: Drinking a glass of water prior to eating might increase feelings of fullness and decrease the desire to overindulge.

12. **Never Take Food Out of the Box or Bag**: Refrain from eating straight out of the package when you are snacking. To help you restrict how much you eat, portion out your snack onto a small dish or plate.

13. **Track Sodium Consumption**: Pay attention to the salt level in processed meals. Increased thirst brought on by high salt levels may lead to bigger meal sizes.

14. **Make sensible goals**: Set attainable goals for portion control. Make little adjustments at first and work your way up to more stringent portion control.

15. **Seek Assistance**: Tell your loved ones about your portion control objectives to get their support. They can support you in adhering to your dietary guidelines.

It takes time and consistency to become an expert at portion management when following a renal diet. You may better manage your renal health and dietary limitations by using these tactics and developing portion management as a habit, which will eventually enhance your overall well-being.

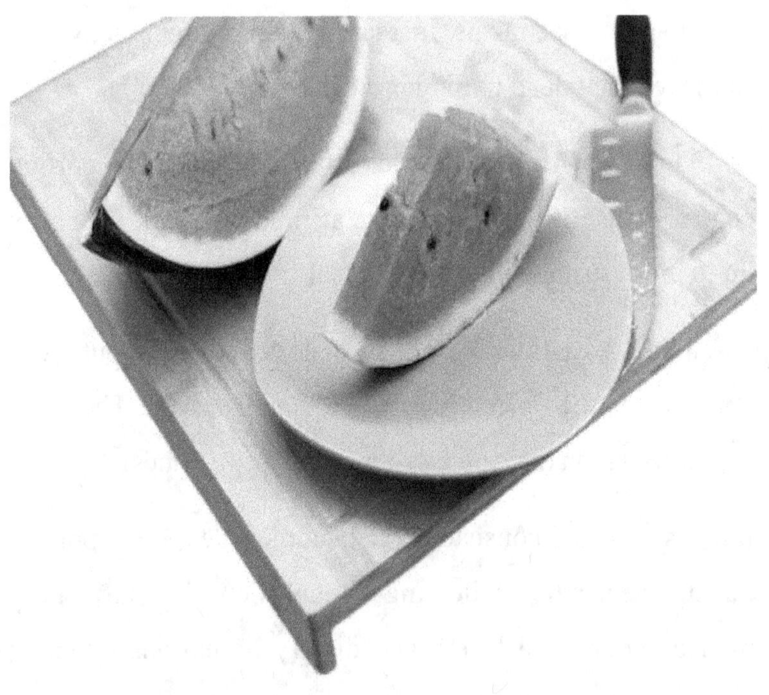

CHAPTER TEN

Conclusion

In summary, starting a renal diet is an admirable initiative to maintain and improve kidney health. The journey may be difficult, but it is characterized by fortitude, flexibility, and an unwavering dedication to well-being.

A renal diet is more than simply limiting; it's also an opportunity to enjoy the variety of foods that are good for your kidneys, try new flavors, and be creative in the kitchen. It's a voyage supported by information and enabled by well-informed decisions.

In my capacity as a dietitian, I urge you to welcome this adventure with open arms and the understanding that you are making significant progress in taking care of your kidneys. Your nutritionist and healthcare provider's advice will be your guide along your journey, so don't forget to periodically check with them.

You may live a more balanced and healthy life by following the renal diet provided you take the proper approach. The trip is worthwhile, and the reward is a better quality of life and kidney health at its peak.

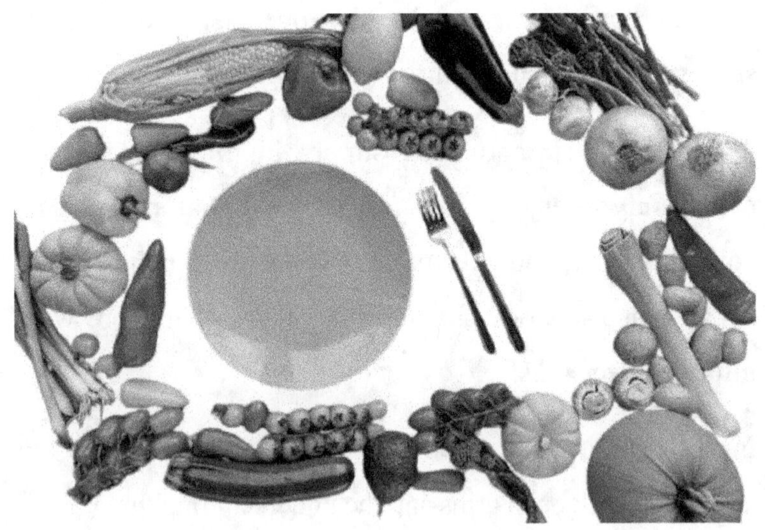

MEAL PLANNER

WEEKLY MEAL PLANNER

			GROCERY LIST
SUNDAY	BREAKFAST		
	LUNCH		
	DINNER		
MONDAY	BREAKFAST		
	LUNCH		
	DINNER		
TUESDAY	BREAKFAST		
	LUNCH		
	DINNER		
WEDNESDAY	BREAKFAST		
	LUNCH		
	DINNER		
THURSDAY	BREAKFAST		SNACKS
	LUNCH		
	DINNER		
FRIDAY	BREAKFAST		
	LUNCH		
	DINNER		
SATURDAY	BREAKFAST		
	LUNCH		
	DINNER		

WEEKLY MEAL PLANNER

SUNDAY	BREAKFAST	
	LUNCH	
	DINNER	
MONDAY	BREAKFAST	
	LUNCH	
	DINNER	
TUESDAY	BREAKFAST	
	LUNCH	
	DINNER	
WEDNESDAY	BREAKFAST	
	LUNCH	
	DINNER	
THURSDAY	BREAKFAST	
	LUNCH	
	DINNER	
FRIDAY	BREAKFAST	
	LUNCH	
	DINNER	
SATURDAY	BREAKFAST	
	LUNCH	
	DINNER	

GROCERY LIST

SNACKS

WEEKLY MEAL PLANNER

				GROCERY LIST
SUNDAY	BREAKFAST			
	LUNCH			
	DINNER			
MONDAY	BREAKFAST			
	LUNCH			
	DINNER			
TUESDAY	BREAKFAST			
	LUNCH			
	DINNER			
WEDNESDAY	BREAKFAST			
	LUNCH			
	DINNER			
THURSDAY	BREAKFAST			SNACKS
	LUNCH			
	DINNER			
FRIDAY	BREAKFAST			
	LUNCH			
	DINNER			
SATURDAY	BREAKFAST			
	LUNCH			
	DINNER			

WEEKLY MEAL PLANNER

			GROCERY LIST
SUNDAY	BREAKFAST		
	LUNCH		
	DINNER		
MONDAY	BREAKFAST		
	LUNCH		
	DINNER		
TUESDAY	BREAKFAST		
	LUNCH		
	DINNER		
WEDNESDAY	BREAKFAST		
	LUNCH		
	DINNER		
THURSDAY	BREAKFAST		SNACKS
	LUNCH		
	DINNER		
FRIDAY	BREAKFAST		
	LUNCH		
	DINNER		
SATURDAY	BREAKFAST		
	LUNCH		
	DINNER		

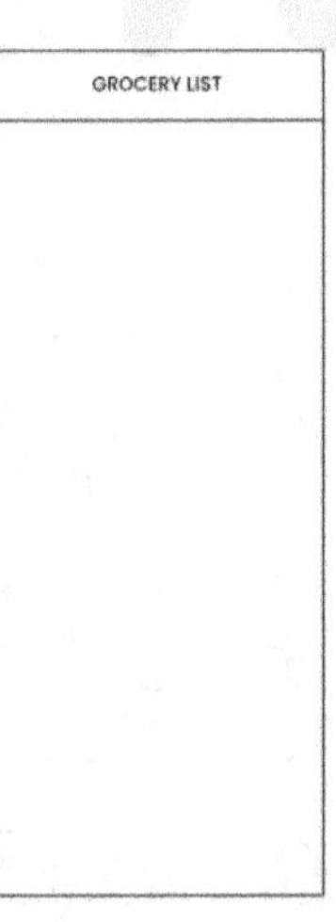
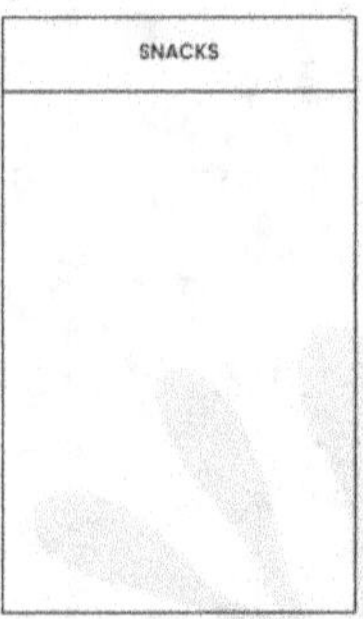

WEEKLY MEAL PLANNER

				GROCERY LIST
SUNDAY	BREAKFAST			
	LUNCH			
	DINNER			
MONDAY	BREAKFAST			
	LUNCH			
	DINNER			
TUESDAY	BREAKFAST			
	LUNCH			
	DINNER			
WEDNESDAY	BREAKFAST			
	LUNCH			
	DINNER			
THURSDAY	BREAKFAST			SNACKS
	LUNCH			
	DINNER			
FRIDAY	BREAKFAST			
	LUNCH			
	DINNER			
SATURDAY	BREAKFAST			
	LUNCH			
	DINNER			

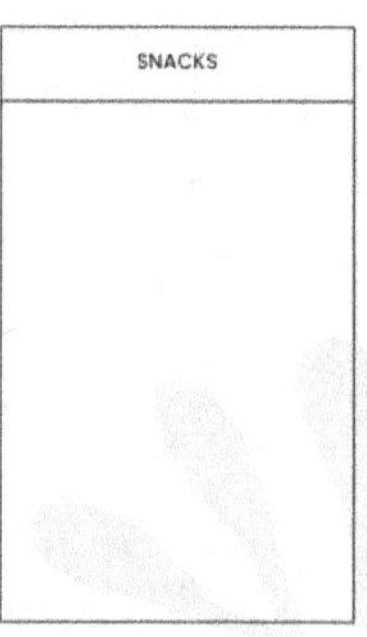

WEEKLY MEAL PLANNER

SUNDAY	BREAKFAST	
	LUNCH	
	DINNER	
MONDAY	BREAKFAST	
	LUNCH	
	DINNER	
TUESDAY	BREAKFAST	
	LUNCH	
	DINNER	
WEDNESDAY	BREAKFAST	
	LUNCH	
	DINNER	
THURSDAY	BREAKFAST	
	LUNCH	
	DINNER	
FRIDAY	BREAKFAST	
	LUNCH	
	DINNER	
SATURDAY	BREAKFAST	
	LUNCH	
	DINNER	

GROCERY LIST

SNACKS

WEEKLY MEAL PLANNER

			GROCERY LIST
SUNDAY	BREAKFAST		
	LUNCH		
	DINNER		
MONDAY	BREAKFAST		
	LUNCH		
	DINNER		
TUESDAY	BREAKFAST		
	LUNCH		
	DINNER		
WEDNESDAY	BREAKFAST		
	LUNCH		
	DINNER		
THURSDAY	BREAKFAST		SNACKS
	LUNCH		
	DINNER		
FRIDAY	BREAKFAST		
	LUNCH		
	DINNER		
SATURDAY	BREAKFAST		
	LUNCH		
	DINNER		

WEEKLY MEAL PLANNER

SUNDAY	BREAKFAST	
	LUNCH	
	DINNER	
MONDAY	BREAKFAST	
	LUNCH	
	DINNER	
TUESDAY	BREAKFAST	
	LUNCH	
	DINNER	
WEDNESDAY	BREAKFAST	
	LUNCH	
	DINNER	
THURSDAY	BREAKFAST	
	LUNCH	
	DINNER	
FRIDAY	BREAKFAST	
	LUNCH	
	DINNER	
SATURDAY	BREAKFAST	
	LUNCH	
	DINNER	

GROCERY LIST

SNACKS

WEEKLY MEAL PLANNER

SUNDAY	BREAKFAST	
	LUNCH	
	DINNER	
MONDAY	BREAKFAST	
	LUNCH	
	DINNER	
TUESDAY	BREAKFAST	
	LUNCH	
	DINNER	
WEDNESDAY	BREAKFAST	
	LUNCH	
	DINNER	
THURSDAY	BREAKFAST	
	LUNCH	
	DINNER	
FRIDAY	BREAKFAST	
	LUNCH	
	DINNER	
SATURDAY	BREAKFAST	
	LUNCH	
	DINNER	

GROCERY LIST

SNACKS

WEEKLY MEAL PLANNER

SUNDAY	BREAKFAST	
	LUNCH	
	DINNER	
MONDAY	BREAKFAST	
	LUNCH	
	DINNER	
TUESDAY	BREAKFAST	
	LUNCH	
	DINNER	
WEDNESDAY	BREAKFAST	
	LUNCH	
	DINNER	
THURSDAY	BREAKFAST	
	LUNCH	
	DINNER	
FRIDAY	BREAKFAST	
	LUNCH	
	DINNER	
SATURDAY	BREAKFAST	
	LUNCH	
	DINNER	

GROCERY LIST

SNACKS

WEEKLY MEAL PLANNER

SUNDAY	BREAKFAST		
	LUNCH		
	DINNER		
MONDAY	BREAKFAST		
	LUNCH		
	DINNER		
TUESDAY	BREAKFAST		
	LUNCH		
	DINNER		
WEDNESDAY	BREAKFAST		
	LUNCH		
	DINNER		
THURSDAY	BREAKFAST		
	LUNCH		
	DINNER		
FRIDAY	BREAKFAST		
	LUNCH		
	DINNER		
SATURDAY	BREAKFAST		
	LUNCH		
	DINNER		

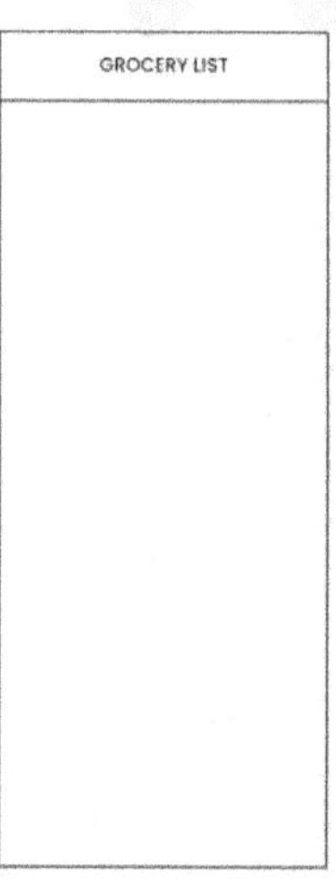

GROCERY LIST

SNACKS

WEEKLY MEAL PLANNER

				GROCERY LIST
SUNDAY	BREAKFAST			
	LUNCH			
	DINNER			
MONDAY	BREAKFAST			
	LUNCH			
	DINNER			
TUESDAY	BREAKFAST			
	LUNCH			
	DINNER			
WEDNESDAY	BREAKFAST			
	LUNCH			
	DINNER			
THURSDAY	BREAKFAST			
	LUNCH			SNACKS
	DINNER			
FRIDAY	BREAKFAST			
	LUNCH			
	DINNER			
SATURDAY	BREAKFAST			
	LUNCH			
	DINNER			

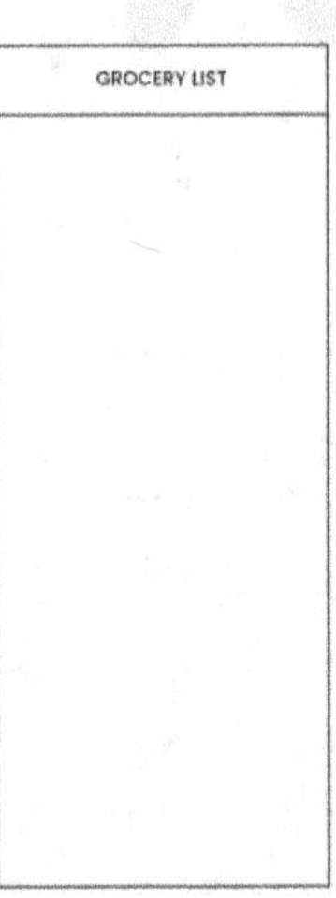

WEEKLY MEAL PLANNER

SUNDAY	BREAKFAST	
	LUNCH	
	DINNER	
MONDAY	BREAKFAST	
	LUNCH	
	DINNER	
TUESDAY	BREAKFAST	
	LUNCH	
	DINNER	
WEDNESDAY	BREAKFAST	
	LUNCH	
	DINNER	
THURSDAY	BREAKFAST	
	LUNCH	
	DINNER	
FRIDAY	BREAKFAST	
	LUNCH	
	DINNER	
SATURDAY	BREAKFAST	
	LUNCH	
	DINNER	

GROCERY LIST

SNACKS

WEEKLY MEAL PLANNER

SUNDAY	BREAKFAST	
	LUNCH	
	DINNER	
MONDAY	BREAKFAST	
	LUNCH	
	DINNER	
TUESDAY	BREAKFAST	
	LUNCH	
	DINNER	
WEDNESDAY	BREAKFAST	
	LUNCH	
	DINNER	
THURSDAY	BREAKFAST	
	LUNCH	
	DINNER	
FRIDAY	BREAKFAST	
	LUNCH	
	DINNER	
SATURDAY	BREAKFAST	
	LUNCH	
	DINNER	

GROCERY LIST

SNACKS

WEEKLY MEAL PLANNER

			GROCERY LIST
SUNDAY	BREAKFAST		
	LUNCH		
	DINNER		
MONDAY	BREAKFAST		
	LUNCH		
	DINNER		
TUESDAY	BREAKFAST		
	LUNCH		
	DINNER		
WEDNESDAY	BREAKFAST		
	LUNCH		
	DINNER		
THURSDAY	BREAKFAST		
	LUNCH		
	DINNER	SNACKS
FRIDAY	BREAKFAST		
	LUNCH		
	DINNER		
SATURDAY	BREAKFAST		
	LUNCH		
	DINNER		

WEEKLY MEAL PLANNER

			GROCERY LIST
SUNDAY	BREAKFAST		
	LUNCH		
	DINNER		
MONDAY	BREAKFAST		
	LUNCH		
	DINNER		
TUESDAY	BREAKFAST		
	LUNCH		
	DINNER		
WEDNESDAY	BREAKFAST		
	LUNCH		
	DINNER		
THURSDAY	BREAKFAST		SNACKS
	LUNCH		
	DINNER		
FRIDAY	BREAKFAST		
	LUNCH		
	DINNER		
SATURDAY	BREAKFAST		
	LUNCH		
	DINNER		

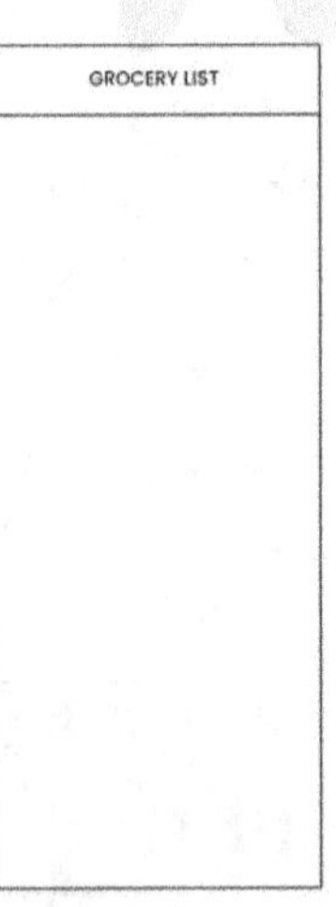
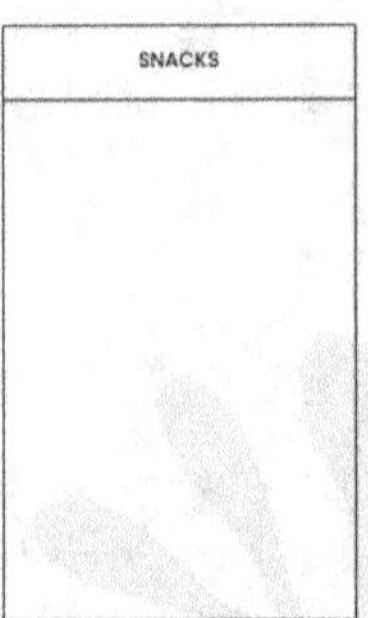

WEEKLY MEAL PLANNER

SUNDAY	BREAKFAST	
	LUNCH	
	DINNER	
MONDAY	BREAKFAST	
	LUNCH	
	DINNER	
TUESDAY	BREAKFAST	
	LUNCH	
	DINNER	
WEDNESDAY	BREAKFAST	
	LUNCH	
	DINNER	
THURSDAY	BREAKFAST	
	LUNCH	
	DINNER	
FRIDAY	BREAKFAST	
	LUNCH	
	DINNER	
SATURDAY	BREAKFAST	
	LUNCH	
	DINNER	

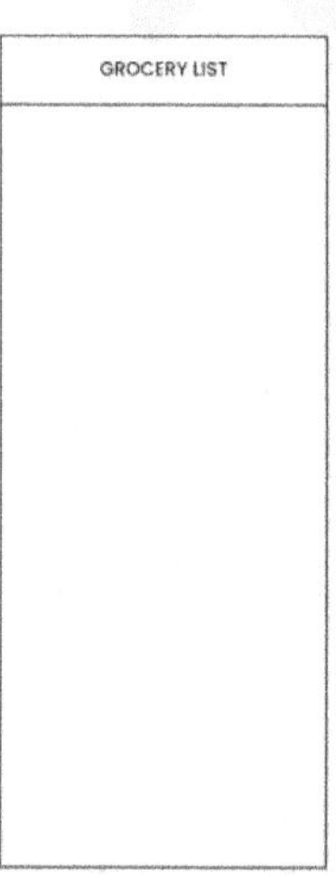

GROCERY LIST

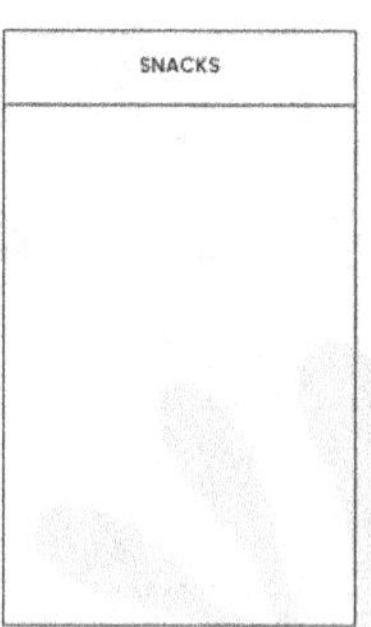

SNACKS

WEEKLY MEAL PLANNER

SUNDAY	BREAKFAST	
	LUNCH	
	DINNER	
MONDAY	BREAKFAST	
	LUNCH	
	DINNER	
TUESDAY	BREAKFAST	
	LUNCH	
	DINNER	
WEDNESDAY	BREAKFAST	
	LUNCH	
	DINNER	
THURSDAY	BREAKFAST	
	LUNCH	
	DINNER	
FRIDAY	BREAKFAST	
	LUNCH	
	DINNER	
SATURDAY	BREAKFAST	
	LUNCH	
	DINNER	

GROCERY LIST

SNACKS

WEEKLY MEAL PLANNER

SUNDAY	BREAKFAST	
	LUNCH	
	DINNER	
MONDAY	BREAKFAST	
	LUNCH	
	DINNER	
TUESDAY	BREAKFAST	
	LUNCH	
	DINNER	
WEDNESDAY	BREAKFAST	
	LUNCH	
	DINNER	
THURSDAY	BREAKFAST	
	LUNCH	
	DINNER	
FRIDAY	BREAKFAST	
	LUNCH	
	DINNER	
SATURDAY	BREAKFAST	
	LUNCH	
	DINNER	

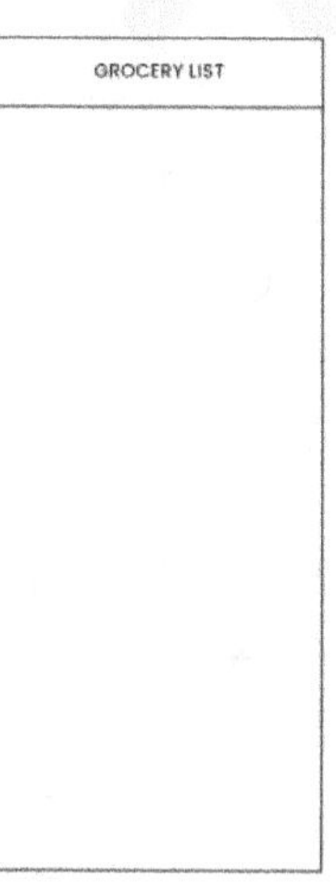

GROCERY LIST

SNACKS

WEEKLY MEAL PLANNER

SUNDAY	BREAKFAST	
	LUNCH	
	DINNER	
MONDAY	BREAKFAST	
	LUNCH	
	DINNER	
TUESDAY	BREAKFAST	
	LUNCH	
	DINNER	
WEDNESDAY	BREAKFAST	
	LUNCH	
	DINNER	
THURSDAY	BREAKFAST	
	LUNCH	
	DINNER	
FRIDAY	BREAKFAST	
	LUNCH	
	DINNER	
SATURDAY	BREAKFAST	
	LUNCH	
	DINNER	

GROCERY LIST

SNACKS

WEEKLY MEAL PLANNER

			GROCERY LIST
SUNDAY	BREAKFAST		
	LUNCH		
	DINNER		
MONDAY	BREAKFAST		
	LUNCH		
	DINNER		
TUESDAY	BREAKFAST		
	LUNCH		
	DINNER		
WEDNESDAY	BREAKFAST		
	LUNCH		
	DINNER		
THURSDAY	BREAKFAST		SNACKS
	LUNCH		
	DINNER		
FRIDAY	BREAKFAST		
	LUNCH		
	DINNER		
SATURDAY	BREAKFAST		
	LUNCH		
	DINNER		

WEEKLY MEAL PLANNER

SUNDAY	BREAKFAST	
	LUNCH	
	DINNER	
MONDAY	BREAKFAST	
	LUNCH	
	DINNER	
TUESDAY	BREAKFAST	
	LUNCH	
	DINNER	
WEDNESDAY	BREAKFAST	
	LUNCH	
	DINNER	
THURSDAY	BREAKFAST	
	LUNCH	
	DINNER	
FRIDAY	BREAKFAST	
	LUNCH	
	DINNER	
SATURDAY	BREAKFAST	
	LUNCH	
	DINNER	

GROCERY LIST

SNACKS

WEEKLY MEAL PLANNER

SUNDAY	BREAKFAST	
	LUNCH	
	DINNER	
MONDAY	BREAKFAST	
	LUNCH	
	DINNER	
TUESDAY	BREAKFAST	
	LUNCH	
	DINNER	
WEDNESDAY	BREAKFAST	
	LUNCH	
	DINNER	
THURSDAY	BREAKFAST	
	LUNCH	
	DINNER	
FRIDAY	BREAKFAST	
	LUNCH	
	DINNER	
SATURDAY	BREAKFAST	
	LUNCH	
	DINNER	

GROCERY LIST

SNACKS

WEEKLY MEAL PLANNER

SUNDAY	BREAKFAST	
	LUNCH	
	DINNER	
MONDAY	BREAKFAST	
	LUNCH	
	DINNER	
TUESDAY	BREAKFAST	
	LUNCH	
	DINNER	
WEDNESDAY	BREAKFAST	
	LUNCH	
	DINNER	
THURSDAY	BREAKFAST	
	LUNCH	
	DINNER	
FRIDAY	BREAKFAST	
	LUNCH	
	DINNER	
SATURDAY	BREAKFAST	
	LUNCH	
	DINNER	

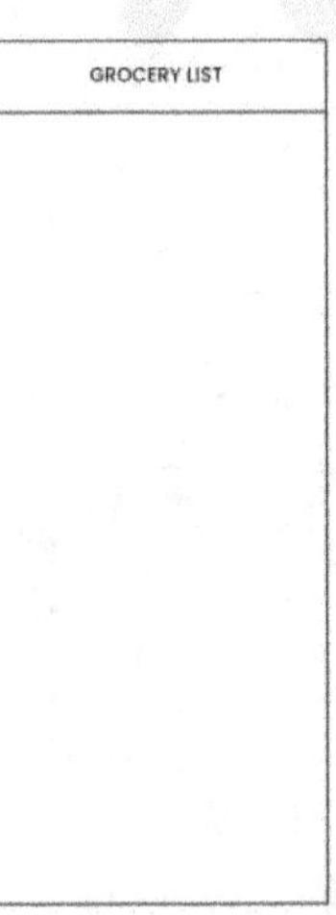

GROCERY LIST

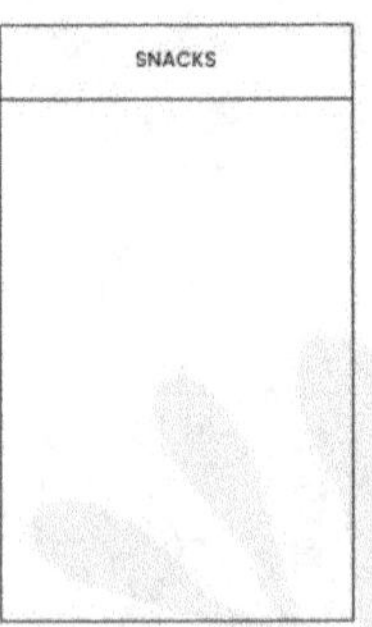

SNACKS

WEEKLY MEAL PLANNER

			GROCERY LIST
SUNDAY	BREAKFAST		
	LUNCH		
	DINNER		
MONDAY	BREAKFAST		
	LUNCH		
	DINNER		
TUESDAY	BREAKFAST		
	LUNCH		
	DINNER		
WEDNESDAY	BREAKFAST		
	LUNCH		
	DINNER		
THURSDAY	BREAKFAST		SNACKS
	LUNCH		
	DINNER		
FRIDAY	BREAKFAST		
	LUNCH		
	DINNER		
SATURDAY	BREAKFAST		
	LUNCH		
	DINNER		

WEEKLY MEAL PLANNER

SUNDAY	BREAKFAST	
	LUNCH	
	DINNER	
MONDAY	BREAKFAST	
	LUNCH	
	DINNER	
TUESDAY	BREAKFAST	
	LUNCH	
	DINNER	
WEDNESDAY	BREAKFAST	
	LUNCH	
	DINNER	
THURSDAY	BREAKFAST	
	LUNCH	
	DINNER	
FRIDAY	BREAKFAST	
	LUNCH	
	DINNER	
SATURDAY	BREAKFAST	
	LUNCH	
	DINNER	

GROCERY LIST

SNACKS

WEEKLY MEAL PLANNER

			GROCERY LIST
SUNDAY	BREAKFAST		
	LUNCH		
	DINNER		
MONDAY	BREAKFAST		
	LUNCH		
	DINNER		
TUESDAY	BREAKFAST		
	LUNCH		
	DINNER		
WEDNESDAY	BREAKFAST		
	LUNCH		
	DINNER		
THURSDAY	BREAKFAST		
	LUNCH		
	DINNER	SNACKS
FRIDAY	BREAKFAST		
	LUNCH		
	DINNER		
SATURDAY	BREAKFAST		
	LUNCH		
	DINNER		

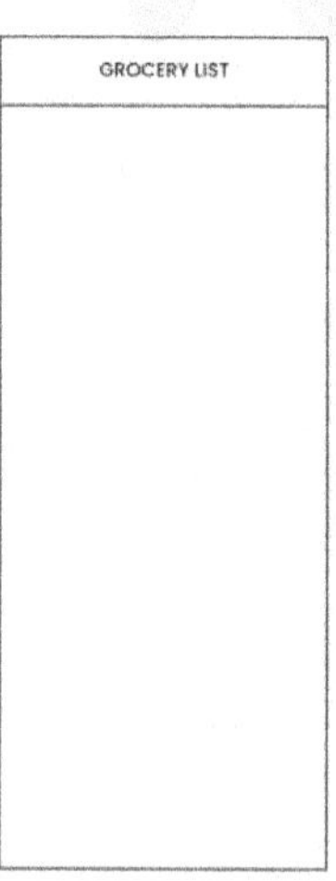

WEEKLY MEAL PLANNER

SUNDAY	BREAKFAST	
	LUNCH	
	DINNER	
MONDAY	BREAKFAST	
	LUNCH	
	DINNER	
TUESDAY	BREAKFAST	
	LUNCH	
	DINNER	
WEDNESDAY	BREAKFAST	
	LUNCH	
	DINNER	
THURSDAY	BREAKFAST	
	LUNCH	
	DINNER	
FRIDAY	BREAKFAST	
	LUNCH	
	DINNER	
SATURDAY	BREAKFAST	
	LUNCH	
	DINNER	

GROCERY LIST

SNACKS

WEEKLY MEAL PLANNER

			GROCERY LIST
SUNDAY	BREAKFAST		
	LUNCH		
	DINNER		
MONDAY	BREAKFAST		
	LUNCH		
	DINNER		
TUESDAY	BREAKFAST		
	LUNCH		
	DINNER		
WEDNESDAY	BREAKFAST		
	LUNCH		
	DINNER		
THURSDAY	BREAKFAST		SNACKS
	LUNCH		
	DINNER		
FRIDAY	BREAKFAST		
	LUNCH		
	DINNER		
SATURDAY	BREAKFAST		
	LUNCH		
	DINNER		

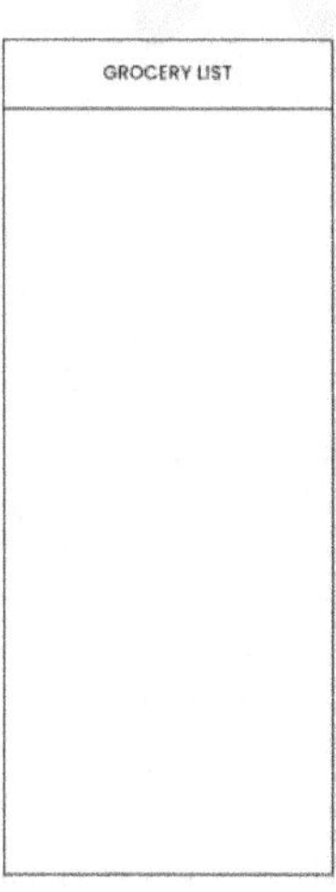

WEEKLY MEAL PLANNER

			GROCERY LIST
SUNDAY	BREAKFAST		
	LUNCH		
	DINNER		
MONDAY	BREAKFAST		
	LUNCH		
	DINNER		
TUESDAY	BREAKFAST		
	LUNCH		
	DINNER		
WEDNESDAY	BREAKFAST		
	LUNCH		
	DINNER		
THURSDAY	BREAKFAST		SNACKS
	LUNCH		
	DINNER		
FRIDAY	BREAKFAST		
	LUNCH		
	DINNER		
SATURDAY	BREAKFAST		
	LUNCH		
	DINNER